ABC OF DERMATOLOGY

ABC OF DERMATOLOGY

PAUL K BUXTON FRCPED, FRCPC

Consultant dermatologist
Royal Infirmary, Edinburgh, and Fife Health Board

with contributions from
D J GAWKRODGER, D W S HARRIS,
D KEMMETT, A L WRIGHT

Articles published in
the *British Medical Journal*

Published by the British Medical Association
Tavistock Square, London WC1H 9JR

© British Medical Journal 1988

First published 1988
Reprinted 1989
Reprinted 1990

British Library Cataloguing in Publication Data

Buxton, P K
    ABC of dermatology.
    1. Medicine. Dermatology
    I. Title   II. Gawkrodger, David J
    III. British Medical Association
    IV. British Medical Journal: 0007-1447
    616.5

ISBN 0-7279-0220-2

Printed in Great Britain by Jolly & Barber Ltd, Rugby
Typesetting by Bedford Typesetters Ltd, Bedford

Contents

INTRODUCTION

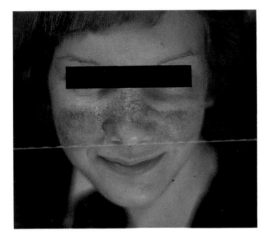

Lupus erythematosus.

The object of this series is to provide the non-specialist with a practical guide to the diagnosis and treatment of skin conditions. Instead of the usual systematic description of each individual disease, the history, clinical appearance, and pathology of a few common key conditions are discussed. These are used as a basis for comparison with other skin diseases.

This approach is suitable for most types of skin lesion that present as rashes, blisters, or ulcers, for example. Some subjects such as allergic reactions, autoimmunity, acne, and infections, however, are covered in a more conventional didactic manner.

One advantage of dealing with dermatological conditions is that nature presents us with the lesion to examine and interpret without the need for complex investigations, although a biopsy is sometimes needed to make or confirm the diagnosis. An understanding of the histological changes underlying the clinical presentation makes the interpretation of skin lesions easier and more interesting. Consequently, clinical descriptions are accompanied by an account of the underlying pathological processes.

Many skin diseases reflect pathological processes in other organs and indeed may be the first sign of disease. For example, a girl presented recently with a rash on her face suggestive of lupus erythematosus and a history of lassitude, weight loss, and weakness. The diagnosis of lupus erythematosus with renal disease was confirmed on subsequent investigation. Such dermatological connections with systemic disease are mentioned in the relevant places.

Descriptive terms

All specialties have their own common terms, and familiarity with a few of those used in dermatology is a great help. The most important are defined below.

Macule

Derived from the Latin for a stain, the term macule is used to describe changes in colour or consistency without any elevation above the surface of the surrounding skin. There may be an increase of melanin, giving a black or blue colour depending on the depth of the pigment. Loss of melanin leads to a white macule. Vascular dilatation and inflammation produce erythema.

Epidermis

Dermis

Macule
(a) Melanin pigment *in* epidermis.
(b) Melanin pigment *below* epidermis.
(c) Erythema due to dilated dermal blood vessels.
(d) Inflammation in dermis.

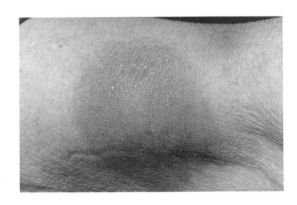

Introduction

Papules and nodules

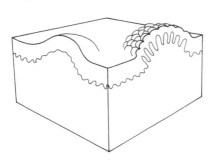

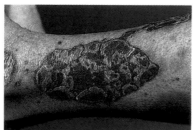

15mm

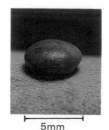

5mm

A papule is a circumscribed, raised lesion, conventionally less than 1 cm in diameter. It may be due to either epidermal or dermal changes.

A nodule is similar to a papule but over 1 cm in diameter.

Plaque

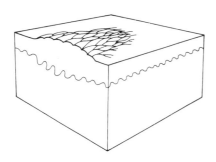

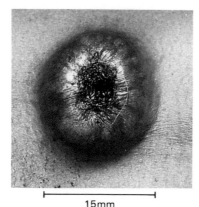

Plaque is one of those terms which convey a clear meaning to dermatologists but is often not understood by others. To take it literally, one can think of a commemorative plaque stuck on the wall of a building with a large area relative to its height and a well defined edge. Plaques are most commonly seen in psoriasis.

Vesicles and bullae

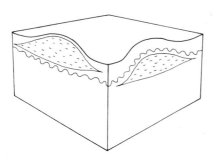

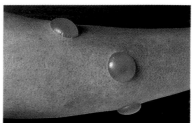

Vesicles and bullae are raised lesions that contain fluid. A bulla is a vesicle larger than 0·5 cm. They may be superficial within the epidermis or situated in the dermis below it.

Lichenification

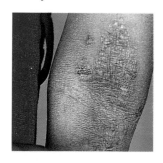

Lichenification is another term frequently used in dermatology as a relic of the days of purely descriptive medicine. Some resemblance to lichen seen on rocks and trees does occur, with hard thickening of the skin and accentuated skin markings. It is most often seen as a result of prolonged rubbing of the skin in localised areas of eczema.

Nummular lesions

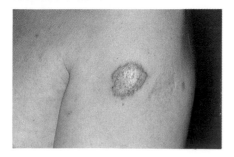

The word nummular literally means a "coin like" lesion. There is no hard and fast distinction from *discoid* lesions, which are flat disc like lesions of variable size. It is most often used to describe a type of eczematous lesion.

Pustules

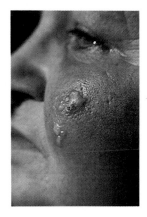

The term pustule is applied to lesions containing purulent material—which may be due to infection, as in the case shown, or sterile pustules are seen in pustular psoriasis.

Rashes

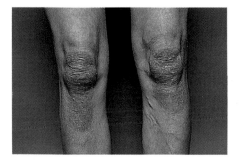

Psoriasis of both legs.

A simplistic but helpful approach to rashes is to classify them as coming from "inside" or "outside." Examples of inside, or endogenous, rashes are atopic eczema and drug rashes, whereas fungal infections or contact dermatitis are from outside. Each type has its own distinctive characteristics.

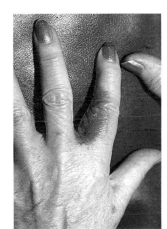

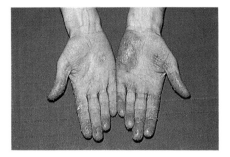

Symmetrical rash—irritant dermatitis.

Asymmetrical rash—contact dermatitis.

Symmetry

Most endogenous rashes affect both sides of the body: think of the atopic child or man with psoriasis on his knees. Of course, not all exogenous rashes are asymmetrical. A seamstress uses scissors in her right hand, where she develops allergy to metal, but a hairdresser or nurse can develop contact dermatitis on both hands.

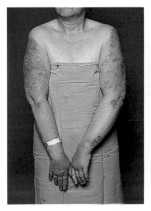
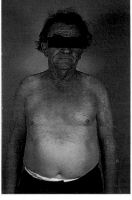

Allergic reactions producing photosensitivity.

Distribution

It is useful to be aware of the usual sites of common skin conditions. These are shown in the appropriate sections. Eruptions that appear only on areas exposed to sun may, of course, be entirely or partially due to sunlight. Some conditions are due to a sensitivity to sunlight alone, such as polymorphous light eruption, or a photosensitivity to topically applied substances or drugs taken internally.

Introduction

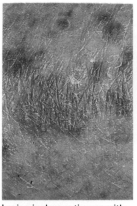

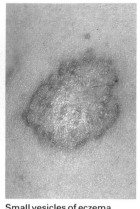

Lesion in deeper tissues with normal epidermis.

Small vesicles of eczema.

Morphology

The appearance of skin lesions gives several clues to the pathological processes.

The surface may consist of normal epidermis overlying a lesion in the deeper tissues. This is characteristic of many types of erythema in which there is dilatation of the dermal vessels with associated inflammation or vasculitis. However, the epidermis may be abnormal. For example, increasing thickness of the keratin layer may form scales, as in psoriasis, or a more uniform thickening in areas lichenified by rubbing. An eczematous process is characterised by both scaling and small vesicles forming in the epidermis.

The margin of some lesions is very well defined, as in psoriasis or lichen planus, but in eczema it merges into normal skin.

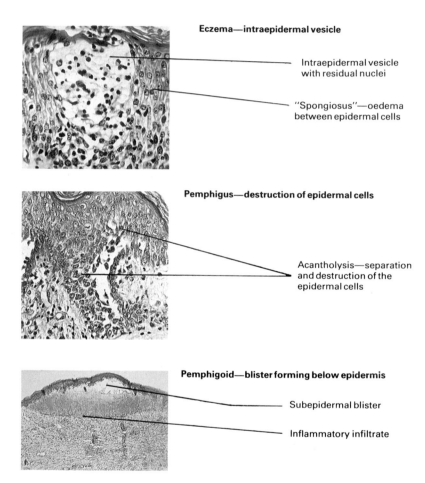

Eczema—intraepidermal vesicle

Intraepidermal vesicle with residual nuclei

"Spongiosus"—oedema between epidermal cells

Pemphigus—destruction of epidermal cells

Acantholysis—separation and destruction of the epidermal cells

Pemphigoid—blister forming below epidermis

Subepidermal blister

Inflammatory infiltrate

Blisters or vesicles occur as a result of (*a*) oedema between the epidermal cells or (*b*) destruction of epidermal cells or (*c*) the result of separation of the epidermis from the deeper tissues. Of course, more than one mechanism may occur in the same lesion. Oedema within the epidermis is seen in endogenous eczema, although it may not be apparent clinically, particularly if it is overshadowed by inflammation and scaling. It is also a feature of contact dermatitis. Widespread blisters occur in:

(*a*) viral diseases such as chickenpox; hand, foot, and mouth disease; and herpes simplex;

(*b*) bacterial infections such as impetigo; and

(*c*) primary blistering disorders such as dermatitis herpetiformis, pemphigus, and pemphigoid and metabolic disorders such as porphyria.

Bullae may occur in congenital conditions (such as epidermolysis bullosa), lichen planus, and pemphigoid without much inflammation. On the other hand, those forming as a result of vasculitis, sunburn, or an allergic reaction may be associated with pronounced inflammation. In pustular psoriasis there are deeper pustules, containing polymorphs but sterile, which show little inflammation. Drug rashes can appear as a bullous eruption.

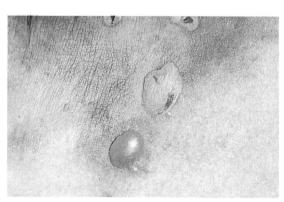

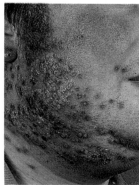

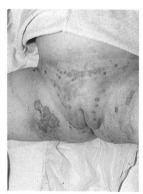

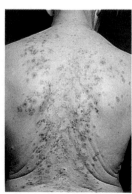

Pemphigus—superficial blister.

Herpes simplex.

Impetigo.

Dermatitis herpetiformis.

Assessment of the patient

A relevant history should be taken with particular reference to:

Where?—Site of initial lesion(s) and subsequent changes in distribution.

When?—Have there been any previous episodes? If so, note the duration of these and the present condition.

Progress?—Is it getting better or worse? Does it itch?

Treatment?—Treatment to date—both by prescription and by home remedies.

What else?—Are there any associated conditions? Ask about any medication and drugs, whether prescribed or bought "over the counter."

We now come to the matter of using these basic concepts in the diagnosis of lesions in practice. In the next four chapters two common skin diseases are considered—psoriasis, which affects 1-2% of the population, and eczema, an even more common complaint. Both are rashes with epidermal changes. The difficulty arises with the unusual lesion: Is it a rarity or a variation of a common disease? What should make us consider further investigation? Is it safe to wait and see if it resolves or persists? The usual clinical presentations of psoriasis and eczema are also used as a basis for comparison with variations of the usual pattern and other skin conditions.

The effect of a skin condition on the patient's life and the patient's attitude to it must always be taken into account. For example, severe pustular psoriasis of the hands can be devastating for a self employed electrician and total hair loss from the scalp very distressing for a 16 year old girl.

Fear that a skin condition may be due to cancer or infection is often present and reassurance should always be given whether asked for or not. If there is the possibility of a serious underlying cause that requires further investigation it is part of good management to answer any questions the patient has and provide an explanation that he can understand. We all forget this aspect of medical practice at times.

PSORIASIS

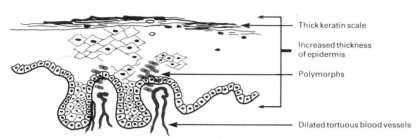

Increased epidermal proliferation—nuclei found . . . throughout the epidermis

Thick keratin scale

Increased thickness of epidermis

Polymorphs

Dilated tortuous blood vessels

The familiar pink or red lesions with a scaling surface and well defined edge are easily recognised. These changes can be related to the histological appearance.

(1) The increased thickness of the epidermis, presence of nuclei above the basal layer, and thick keratin are related to increased epidermal turnover.

(2) Because the epidermis is dividing it does not differentiate adequately into normal keratin scales. These are readily removed to reveal the tortuous blood vessels beneath—clinically, "Auspitz sign." The psoriatic plaque can be likened to a brick wall badly built by a workman in too much of a hurry—it may be high but it is easily knocked down.

(3) The polymorphs that migrate into the epidermis form sterile pustules in pustular psoriasis. These are most commonly seen on the palms and soles.

(4) The dilated blood vessels can be a main feature, giving the clinical picture of intense erythema.

The equivalent changes in the nail cause thickening and "pits" 0·5-1·0 mm in diameter on the surface; these are thought to be due to small areas of psoriatic changes in the upper nail plate that then fall out.

While still considering the individual lesion remember the following points.

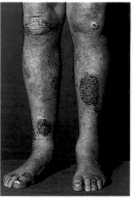 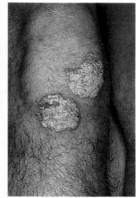

Plaques of psoriasis.

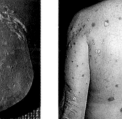 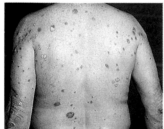 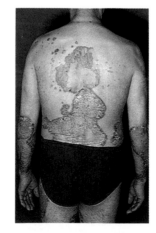

Pitting of nail.

Small and large lesions.

The *size* of the lesions varies from a few millimetres to very extensive plaques.

Scaling may predominate, giving a thick plaque, which is sometimes likened to limpets on the sea shore, hence the name "rupioid." Scratching the surface produces a waxy appearance—the "tache de bougie" (literally "a line of candle wax").

Erythema may be conspicuous, especially in lesions on the trunk and flexures.

Pustules are rare on the trunk and limbs, but deep seated pustules on the palm and soles are fairly common.

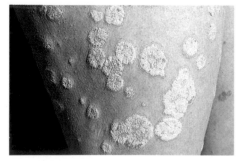 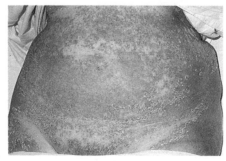 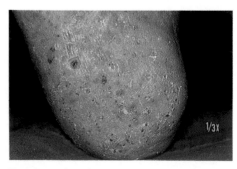

Rupioid lesions.

Widespread pustular psoriasis.

Pustules on the sole.

The typical patient

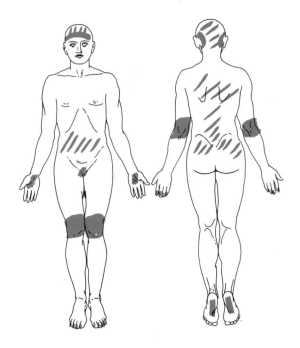

Psoriasis usually occurs in early adult life, but the onset can be at any time from infancy to old age, when the appearance is often atypical. The following factors in the history may help in making a diagnosis.

● There may be a family history.
● The onset can occur after any type of stress, including infection, trauma, or childbirth.
● The lesions may first appear at sites of minor trauma—the Köbner phenomenon.
● The lesions usually clear on exposure to the sun.
● Typically, psoriasis does not itch.
● There may be associated arthropathy—affecting either the fingers and toes or a single large joint.

Clinical presentation

Patients usually present with plaques and sometimes annular lesions on the elbows, knees, and scalp. Patients with psoriasis show the Köbner phenomenon with lesions developing in areas of skin trauma such as scars or minor scratches. Normal everyday trauma such as handling heavy machinery may produce hyperkeratotic lesions on the palms. In the scalp there is scaling, sometimes producing very thick accretions. Erythema often extends beyond the hair margin. The nails show "pits" and also thickening with separation of the nail from the nail bed (onycholysis).

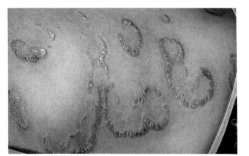

Annular lesions.

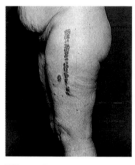

Köbner phenomenon: psoriasis in surgical scar.

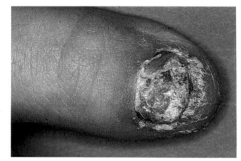

Psoriasis of the nail.

Variations

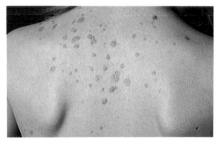

Guttate psoriasis.

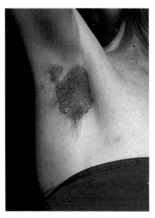

Flexural psoriasis.

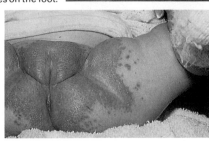

Pustules on the foot.

Napkin psoriasis.

Guttate psoriasis—from the Latin *gutta*, a drop—consists of widespread small pink macules that look like drops of paint. It usually occurs in adolescents and often follows an acute β haemolytic streptococcal infection. There may be much distress to both parent and child when a previously healthy adolescent erupts in apparent leprous spots.

Pustular lesions occur as chronic deep seated lesions on the palms and soles with surrounding erythema which develop a brown colour and scaling. In clinics north of the border these pustules make the patient ask whether the condition is "smitten"—that is, infectious. It is important always to explain that it is not.

Flexural psoriasis produces well defined erythematous areas in the axillae and groins and beneath the breasts. Scaling is minimal or absent.

Napkin psoriasis in children may present with typical psoriatic lesions or a more diffuse erythematous eruption with exudative rather than scaling lesions.

Psoriasis

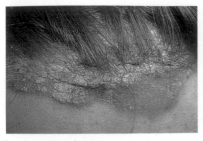

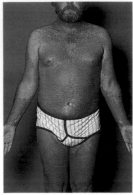

Above: scalp psoriasis. Right: erythrodermic psoriasis.

Generalised pustular psoriasis is uncommon. Superficial pustules develop in an area of intense erythema.

Erythrodermic psoriasis is a serious, even life threatening, condition with erythema affecting nearly the whole of the skin. Diagnosis may not be easy as the characteristic scaling of psoriasis is absent, although this usually precedes the erythroderma. Less commonly the erythema develops suddenly without preceding lesions. There is a considerable increase in cutaneous blood flow, heat loss, metabolism, and water loss.

It is important to distinguish between the stable, chronic, plaque type of psoriasis, which is unlikely to develop exacerbations and which responds to tar, disthranol, and ultraviolet treatment, and the more acute erythematous type, which is unstable and likely to spread rapidly, particularly when irritated by tar, dithranol, or ultraviolet light.

Joint disease in psoriasis

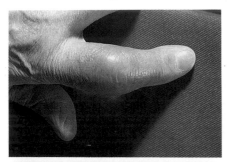

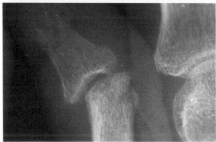

Acute arthropathy.

Patients with seronegative arthropathy of the non-rheumatoid type show double the normal (2%) incidence of psoriasis. Psoriatic arthropathy commonly affects the distal interphalangeal joints, sparing the metacarpophalangeal joints, and is usually asymmetrical. Rheumatoid nodules are absent. The sex ratio is equal but a few patients develop a "rheumatoid like" arthropathy, which is more common in women than in men. There is a third rare group who suffer from arthritic changes, in which there is considerable resorption of bone.

Other members of the families of those with psoriatic arthropathy are affected in 40% of cases.

There may be severe pustular psoriasis of the fingers and toes associated with arthropathy. One patient was so severely affected that she was immobilised until her condition cleared on treatment with methotrexate.

The detailed treatment of psoriasis is covered in the next chapter. The only point to be made here is the importance of encouraging a positive attitude with expectation of improvement but not a permanent cure, since psoriasis can recur at any time. Some patients are unconcerned about very extensive lesions while to others the most minor lesions are a catastrophe.

TREATMENT OF PSORIASIS

Presentation of psoriasis	Treatment of choice	Alternative treatment
Stable plaque	Short contact dithranol	Tar
Extensive stable plaque	PUVA + etretinate	Short contact dithranol
Widespread small plaque	Ultraviolet B	Tar
Guttate psoriasis	Emollients while erupting then ultraviolet B	Weak tar preparations
Facial psoriasis	1% Hydrocortisone ointment	
Flexural psoriasis	Local mild to moderate strength steroids + antifungal	
Pustular psoriasis of hands and feet	Moderate to potent strength local steroid	Etretinate
Acute erythrodermic, unstable, or generalised pustular psoriasis	Inpatient treatment with ichthammol paste. Local steroids may be used in skilled hands	Methotrexate

In deciding on treatment for any individual patient with psoriasis the clinician must take several factors into consideration, including the extent of the disease, the medical and social problems it causes, and the motivation of the patient to treat it. The same degree of disease in two individuals may have very different impacts on their lives depending on their age, marital state, and employment. Thus it is possible only to give guidelines on the correct management of different presentations of psoriasis. The doctor must assess the appropriateness of specific treatments for individuals.

Local treatments

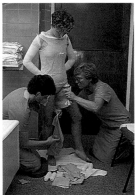
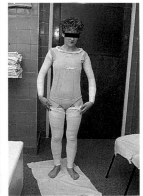
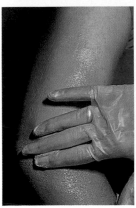
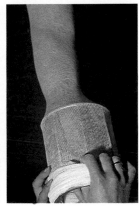

Tar—Crude coal tar has long been used as a safe effective treatment for chronic plaque psoriasis. Its main limitation is its smell and mess, which restrict its use to inpatients, to outpatients who can attend hospital for dressings, or to highly motivated patients with relatively small areas of plaque. Refined preparations of coal tar are cosmetically more acceptable but less effective. Strong coal tar solution can be used in various cream and ointment bases in concentrations of 1 to 10%. The addition of salicylic acid as a keratolytic agent helps to reduce scaling, and a preparation containing 10% strong solution of coal tar, 2% salicylic acid to 100% in Unguentum Merck is an example of a reasonably effective tar preparation which patients often tolerate for home use. The many creams and ointments containing refined coal tar extracts may be useful for treating small, thin plaques of psoriasis but will make little impression on larger, thicker plaques. Guttate psoriasis may well respond to these weaker tar preparations.

Dithranol (or anthralin) is a highly effective synthetic compound, which is now the treatment of choice for chronic plaque psoriasis. Its main problem is its tendency to burn and irritate normal skin. In hospital this is prevented by applying the dithranol in a paste and protecting the surrounding skin with a rim of Vaseline. At home this is difficult to do safely and the recommended regimen for outpatient use is the "short contact method." Here the dithranol is in contact with the skin for a maximum of only 30 minutes, during which it can penetrate the abnormal epidermis over a psoriatic plaque but not the healthy epidermis of normal skin; thus it treats the psoriasis but avoids the burning and irritation. Compliance is excellent as patients do not have to keep the cream on for longer than half an hour a day before their bath or shower. Provided the cautions are noted this is one of the most useful outpatient treatments.

Treatment of psoriasis

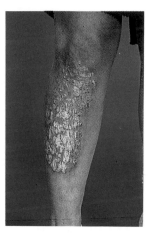

Psoriasis suitable for short contact dithranol treatment.

Bland preparations and emollients—Regular use of an emollient is a simple measure, often forgotten, which may bring much relief from itching and scaling. An emollient should always be used in conjunction with short contact dithranol, and if tar is being used at night an emollient should be used during the day. Suitable emollients are soft white paraffin, Unguentum Merck, or Lipobase. If psoriasis is actively erupting or plaques are hot and inflamed tar or dithranol will not be tolerated, and a bland preparation such as ichthammol paste (1% ichthammol, 15% zinc oxide to 100% in yellow soft paraffin) is the treatment of choice.

Steroids—Steroid creams and ointments do not smell or stain and are pleasant to use. Unfortunately they are not that effective in clearing plaques of psoriasis and the psoriasis tends to rebound after withdrawal, often in a more unstable form. Local steroids are therefore not recommended for chronic plaque psoriasis. Nevertheless, steroids are indicated for certain types of psoriasis. The skin on the face tolerates tar and dithranol poorly, and 1% hydrocortisone ointment is the treatment of choice; more potent steroid preparations should not be used. Flexural psoriasis is another form where tar and dithranol are likely to irritate the skin and steroids are indicated. It is often useful to choose a preparation which combines a mild or moderately potent steroid with an antifungal and antibiotic agent as secondary infection in these warm moist areas is often a problem. Trimovate ointment (clobetasone, oxytetracycline, and nystatin), Canesten HC (hydrocortisone and clotrimazole), and Terra-Cortril Nystatin (hydrocortisone, oxytetracycline, and nystatin) are suitable examples. If the area is very moist an antiseptic paint such as 2% aqueous eosin is a useful if potentially messy addition. If the palms and soles are affected with psoriasis potent steroid ointments such as full strength betamethasone may be indicated. When possible tar paste should be used on top of the steroid at night. Diprosalic ointment combines a potent steroid with salicylic acid and is useful if there is hyperkeratosis. Systemic steroids should *not* be prescribed in psoriasis.

Ultraviolet treatment

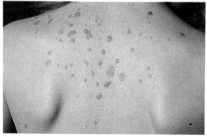

Guttate psoriasis suitable for ultraviolet B treatment.

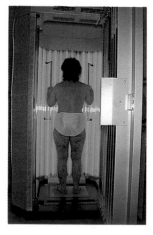

PUVA cabinet.

The two types of ultraviolet radiation used to treat psoriasis are ultraviolet B (290-320 nm), which is effective on its own, and ultraviolet A (320-400 nm), which is little use on its own but effective when used in conjunction with psoralens (PUVA).

Ultraviolet B is indicated for widespread lesions with guttate or small plaque psoriasis in people who can tolerate the sun. It is not particularly effective if the lesions are very thick or bigger than 2·5-5·0 cm in diameter. It should be given by a skilled therapist three times a week with the aim of producing a mild erythema after each treatment. If the dose is increased too quickly painful burning will result; if the increase is too slow the patient will get a good tan rather than effective clearing. When administered correctly a course of ultraviolet B will clear the lesions in five to six weeks.

PUVA should be considered when large plaques of psoriasis affect at least 20% of the surface area of the body. The patient takes methoxsalen (8-methoxypsoralen) two hours before exposure to ultraviolet A. The psoralen (derived from a plant extract) is inactive in the dark but becomes active in the presence of ultraviolet A and interacts with the deoxyribonucleic acid (DNA) in the basal cells of the psoriatic plaques, slowing their growth rate back to normal. Treatment is given three times a week with gradually increasing doses of ultraviolet A, and clearance is usually achieved in five to six weeks. Once the psoriasis has responded the skin can often be kept free of psoriasis by continuing the PUVA once a fortnight or even once every three weeks, but this is not generally recommended in younger patients because of the risks of side effects. High cumulative doses of PUVA are associated with a small increased risk of skin aging, actinic keratosis, squamous cell carcinoma, and basal cell carcinoma. As yet there has been no significantly increased incidence of malignant

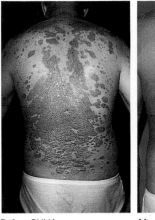 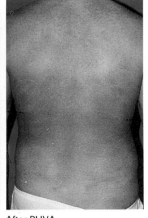

Before PUVA.　　　　　After PUVA.

melanoma among patients treated with PUVA, but PUVA has been available for only about 15 years and this possibility remains a worry. PUVA is therefore an effective treatment for a flare up of psoriasis which is too extensive to manage with local creams at home. It is an alternative to inpatient treatment and usually allows the patient to carry on his or her normal life during treatment. Side effects are almost certainly related to the cumulative amount of PUVA received over the years, and this should be kept as low as possible without denying treatment when indicated.

Systemic treatment

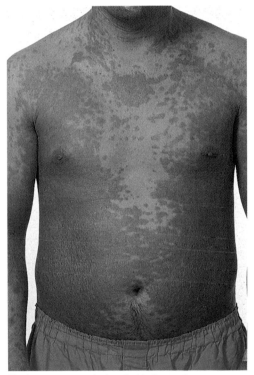

Erythematous psoriasis suitable for methotrexate treatment, having failed to respond to PUVA.

Retinoids—The retinoids are derived from vitamin A, and etretinate, one of the first available, is used to treat psoriasis. Etretinate will thin hyperkeratotic plaques of psoriasis but on its own is not very effective in actually clearing the lesions. It is most commonly used in conjunction with PUVA in a regimen known as Re-PUVA. By combining the two treatments more rapid clearance is achieved with a smaller cumulative dose of PUVA. Maintenance treatment with etretinate prevents relapse after clearance, but its use is not generally recommended because of potential side effects. The main effects are an increase in serum lipid concentrations, disruption of liver function, and the risk of hyperostoses. Etretinate is an unpleasant drug to take, causing dryness of mucous membranes, cracked lips, and peeling of the skin of the palms and soles. It is contraindicated in women of childbearing years because of its known teratogenicity and long half life.

Methotrexate—Occasionally psoriasis fails to respond to any of the treatments discussed so far, and the only way to keep the condition under control is to use methotrexate. A small oral dose (around 10 mg) given once a week is often enough to control the most aggressive psoriasis. The main side effect which limits its use is liver damage and the only reliable method of detecting this early on is by liver biopsy after every cumulative dose of 1·5 g.

Many other drugs have been tried in the treatment of stubborn psoriasis but none have been found to be consistently effective without major side effects. The most recent, which is currently being evaluated, is cyclosporin A. Some dramatic responses have been reported with this drug, but its nephrotoxicity and other side effects will inevitably limit its usefulness.

Scalp psoriasis

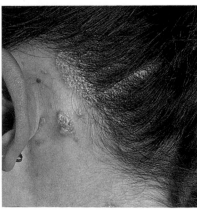

(1) Shampoo regularly with a tar based shampoo such as Polytar or T Gel.

(2) To control thicker scalp psoriasis unresponsive to tar shampoos alone, once or twice a week apply a preparation containing 3% sulphur and 3% salicylic acid in a suitable base and wash it out with a tar shampoo after at least four hours. (The base chosen must balance effectiveness and patient acceptability. Soft white paraffin is effective but extremely hard to wash out. Aqueous cream washes out easily but is not so effective. A good compromise is Unguentum Merck or emulsifying ointment.)

Steroid scalp applications are of limited value but may give some relief if there is a lot of itch and irritation.

Dithranol can be effective in scalp psoriasis but may tint blonde or red hair purple.

ECZEMA AND DERMATITIS

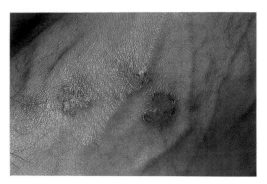

Eczema.

The term eczema covers a wide variety of conditions, from the child with atopic eczema to the adult with an allergy to cement. This leaves "dermatitis" with nothing to its name except being an undefined general term for any type of skin condition. Here I shall use "eczema" to cover endogenous conditions of various types and "contact dermatitis" for those caused by an external agent other than infection. If you tell patients that they have dermatitis they may assume that this is occupational dermatitis. It is not unusual for industrial workers to say, "Is it dermatitis, doctor?"— that is, "Is it due to my job?"

Morphology

Eczema consists of vesicular lesions with erythema and a poorly defined edge. Dryness and scaling then develop. In severe cases it lives up to the literal meaning of eczema, "to boil," with a dense collection of blisters.

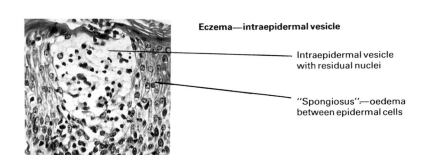

Eczema—intraepidermal vesicle

— Intraepidermal vesicle with residual nuclei

— "Spongiosus"—oedema between epidermal cells

Pathology

Oedema develops between the epidermal cells to form vesicles. The epidermis thickens, with an increase in the keratin layer, while in the dermis there is vasodilatation and an inflammatory infiltrate.

Distribution

The lesions may be generalised, but the following are common patterns.

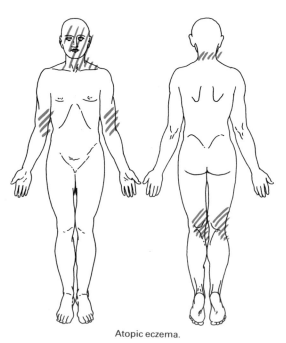

Atopic eczema.

Atopic eczema affects mainly the flexor surfaces of the elbows and knees and the face and neck. To a variable degree it can affect the trunk as well. *Nummular eczema* appears as coin shaped lesions on legs and trunk.

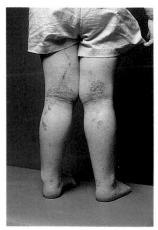

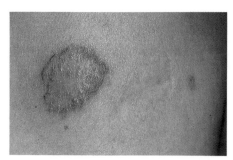

Nummular eczema.

Atopic eczema.

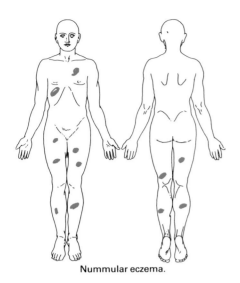

Nummular eczema.

Stasis eczema occurs around the ankles, where there is impaired venous return.

Paget's disease of the breast—While eczema of the nipples and areolae occur in women, any *unilateral*, persistent, area of dermatitis in this region may be due to Paget's disease, in which there is underlying carcinoma of the ducts. In such cases a biopsy is essential.

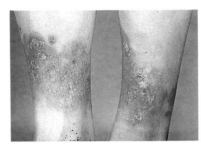

Stasis eczema.

Paget's disease of the nipple.

Atopic eczema

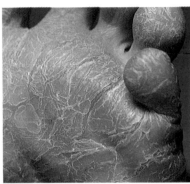

Plantar dermatosis.

The typical patient with atopic eczema is a fretful scratching child with eczema that varies in severity, often from one hour to the next. In the older child or adult eczema is more chronic and widespread and its occurrence is often related to stress. Atopic eczema is common, affecting 3% of all infants, and runs a chronic course with variable remissions. It normally clears during childhood but may continue into adolescence and adult life as a chronic disease. It is often associated with asthma and rhinitis. Sufferers from atopic eczema often have a family history of the condition.

Variants of atopic eczema are pityriasis alba—white patches on the face of children with a fair complexion—and chronic juvenile plantar dermatosis—dry cracked skin of the forefoot in children. This does not affect the interdigital spaces and thus is not due to a fungal infection.

Other types of eczema

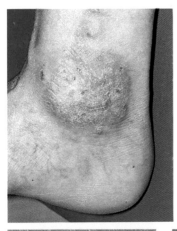

Lichen simplex.

Lichen simplex is a localised area of lichenification produced by rubbing.

Neurodermatitis is a term often used synonymously with lichen simplex. It is also used to describe generalised dryness and itching of the skin, usually in those with atopic eczema.

Asteatotic eczema occurs in older people with a dry, "crazypaving" pattern, particularly on the legs.

Pompholyx is itching vesicles on the fingers, with lesions on the palms and soles in some patients.

Infection can modify the presentation of any type of eczema or contact dermatitis.

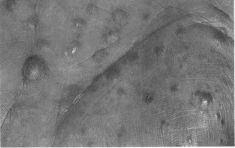

Asteatosis.

Pompholyx.

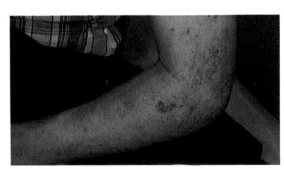

Infected eczema.

13

Eczema and dermatitis
Contact dermatitis

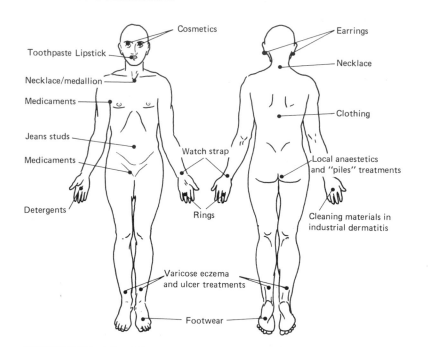

Cosmetics
Toothpaste Lipstick
Necklace/medallion
Medicaments
Jeans studs
Medicaments
Detergents
Watch strap
Rings
Varicose eczema and ulcer treatments
Footwear
Earrings
Necklace
Clothing
Local anaestetics and "piles" treatments
Cleaning materials in industrial dermatitis

Common sources of allergic contact dermatitis	
Jewellery, clothing, wristwatch, scissors, cooking utensils	Nickel—and cobalt occasionally
Cement, leather	Chromate
Hair dyes, tights, shoes	Paraphenylenediamine
Rubber gloves and boots	Rubber preservative chemicals
Creams, ointments, cosmetics	Preservatives (parabenz-quarternium), Balsam of Peru, Fragrances, Lanolin Neomycin, Benzocaine, in medicated ointments

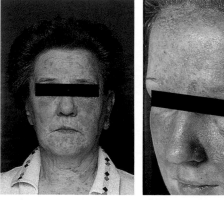

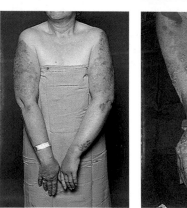

Allergic reactions to: (top left) topical neomycin; (right) dithranol; (bottom left) Solarcaine and sun; and (right) sulphapyridine by mouth.

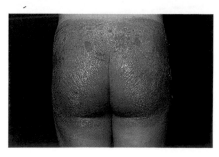

Irritant reaction to bleach.

The skin normally performs its function as a barrier very effectively. If this is overcome by substances penetrating the epidermis an inflammatory response may occur leading to epidermal damage. These changes may be due to either (a) an allergic response to a specific substance acting as a sensitiser or (b) a simple irritant effect. An understanding of the difference between these reactions is helpful in the clinical assessment of contact dermatitis.

The characteristics of allergic dermatitis are (a) previous exposure to the substance concerned; (b) 48 to 96 hours between contact and the development of changes in the skin; (c) activation of previously sensitised sites by contact with the same allergen elsewhere on the body; and (d) persistence of the allergy for many years.

Allergic contact dermatitis can be illustrated by the example of an individual with an allergy to nickel who has previously reacted to a wrist watch. Working with metal objects that contain nickel leads to dermatitis on the hands plus a flare up at the previous site of contact with the watch. The skin clears on holiday but the dermatitis recurs two days after the person returns to work.

On the other hand, *irritant contact dermatitis* has a much less defined clinical course and is caused by a wide variety of substances with no predictable time interval between contact and the appearance of the rash. Dermatitis occurs soon after exposure and the severity varies with the quantity, concentration, and length of exposure to the substance concerned. Previous contact is not required, unlike allergic dermatitis, where previous sensitisation is necessary.

Photodermatitis, caused by the interaction of light and chemical absorbed by the skin, occurs in areas exposed to light. It may be due to (a) drugs taken internally, such as sulphonamides, phenothiazines, and dimethylchlortetracycline, or (b) substances in contact with the skin, such as topical antihistamines, local anaesthetics, cosmetics, and antibacterials.

Morphology—The clinical appearance of both allergic and irritant contact dermatitis may be similar but there are specific changes that help in differentiating them. An acute allergic reaction tends to produce erythema, oedema, and vesicles. The more chronic lesions are often lichenified. Irritant dermatitis may present as slight scaling and itching or extensive epidermal damage resembling a superficial burn, as the child in the illustration shows.

Pathology—The allergic reaction to specific sensitisers leads to a typical eczematous reaction with oedema separating the epidermal cells and blister formation. In irritant dermatitis there may also be eczematous changes but also non-specific inflammation, thickening of keratin, and pyknotic, dead epidermal cells.

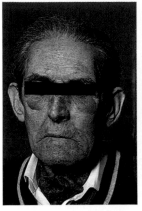
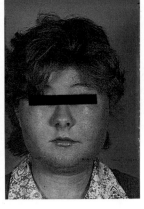
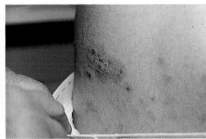

Neomycin
Lanolin (wool alcohol)
Formaldehyde
Tars
Chinaform (the "C" of many
proprietary steroids)

Allergic reactions to: (left) rubber pad on
goggles; (middle) cosmetics; and (above)
elastic in underpants.

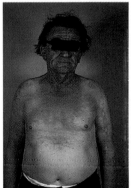
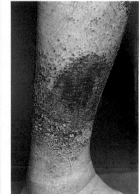

Photodermatitis.   Leg dermatitis.

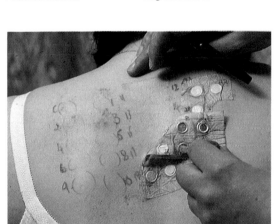

The distribution of the skin changes is often helpful. For example, an itchy rash on the waist may be due to an allergy to rubber in the waistband of underclothing or a metal fastener. Gloves or the rubber lining of goggles can cause a persisting dermatitis. An irritant substance often produces a more diffuse eruption, as shown by the patient who developed itching and redness from dithranol.

Photodermatitis can occur from everyday household substances such as soap—the man in the photograph reacted to the trichlorsalicalanilide in soap he had used before working in his garden. The outline of the area protected by his vest can be seen, and the positive photopatch test is shown below.

An allergy to medications used for treating leg ulcers is a common cause of persisting dermatitis on the leg. Common allergens are listed in the box.

Patch testing

Patch testing is used to determine the substances causing contact dermatitis. The concentration used is critical. If it is too low there may be no reaction, giving a false negative result, and if it is too high it may produce an irritant reaction, which is interpreted as showing an allergy (false positive). Another possible danger is the induction of an allergy by the test substance. The optimum concentration and best vehicle have been found for most common allergens, which are the basis of the "battery" of tests used in most dermatology units.

The test patches are left in place for 48 hours then removed, the sites marked, and any positive reactions noted. A further examination is carried out at 96 hours to detect any further reactions.

It is most important not to put a possible causative substance on the skin in a random manner without proper dilution and without control patches. The results will be meaningless and irritant reactions, which are unpleasant for the patient, may occur.

TREATMENT OF ECZEMA AND INFLAMMATORY DERMATOSES

(1) Treat the patient, not just the rash

(2) Avoid promising complete cure

(3) Be realistic about applying treatments at home

(4) Make sure the patient understands how to carry out the treatment

(5) Advise using emollients and minimal soap

(6) Provide detailed guidance on using steroids

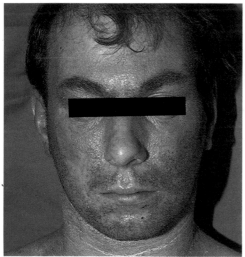

Weeping eczema

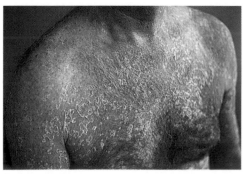

Acute erythema

Treat the patient, not just the rash. Many patients accept their skin condition with equanimity but others suffer much distress—especially if the face and hands are affected. Acceptance by the doctor of the individual and his or her attitudes to the disease goes a long way to helping the patient live with the condition.

The common inflammatory skin diseases can nearly always be improved or cleared—but it is wise not to promise a permanent cure.

Be realistic about the treatment people can apply in their own homes. It is easy to unthinkingly give patients with a widespread rash a large amount of ointment to apply twice daily, which is hardly used because: (a) they have a busy job or young children and simply do not have time to apply ointment to the whole skin; (b) they have arthritic or other limitations of movement and can reach only a small part of the body; (c) the tar or other ointment is smelly or discolours their clothes. Most of us have been guilty of forgetting these factors at one time or another.

Dry skin tends to be itchy, so advise minimal use of soap. Emollients are used to soften the skin, and the simpler the better. Emulsifying ointment *BP* is cheap and effective but rather thick. I advise patients to mix two tablespoons in a kitchen blender with a pint of water—the result is a creamy mixture that can easily be used in the bath. Various proprietary bath oils are available and can be applied directly to wet skin. This is more sensible than putting them in the bath water, which makes the bath slippery with more oil going down the drain than on the skin. There are many proprietary emollients.

Steroid ointments are effective in relieving inflammation and itching but are not always used effectively. Advise patients to use a strong steroid (such as betamethasone or fluocinolone acetonide) frequently for a few days to bring the condition under control; then change to a weaker steroid (dilute betamethasone, fluocinolone, clobetasone, hydrocortisone) less frequently. Strong steroids should not be continued for long periods, and do not prescribe any steroid stronger than hydrocortisone for the face as a rule. Strong steroids can cause atrophy of the skin if used for long periods, particularly when applied under occlusive dressings. On the face they may lead to fluid telangiectasia and acne like pustules. Avoid using steroids on ulcerated areas. Prolonged use of topical steroids may mask an underlying bacterial or fungal infection.

Specific treatment

Wet, inflamed, exuding lesions

(1) Use wet soaks with normal saline or aluminium acetate (0·6%). Potassium permanganate (0·1%) solution should be used if there is any sign of infection.

(2) Use wet compresses rather than dry dressings.

(3) Steroid *creams* should be used as outlined above. Greasy ointment bases just float off on the exudate.

(4) A combined steroid-antibiotic cream is often needed as infection readily develops.

(5) Systemic antibiotics may be required. Take swabs for bacteriological examination first.

Treatment of eczema and inflammatory dermatoses

Dry, scaling, lichenified lesions

(1) Use emollients.

(2) Use steroid *ointments*, with antibiotics if infection is present.

(3) A weak coal tar preparation or ichthammol can be used on top of the ointments. This is particularly useful at night to prevent itching. 1-2% Coal tar can be prescribed in an ointment. For hard, lichenified skin salicylic acid can be incorporated and the following formulation has been found useful in our department: coal tar solution *BP* 10%, salicylic acid 2%, and unguentum drench to 100%. 1% Ichthammol and 15% zinc oxide in white soft paraffin is less likely to irritate than tar and is suitable for childen.

(4) In treating psoriasis start with a weaker tar preparation and progress to a stronger one.

(5) For thick, hyperkeratotic lesions, particularly in the scalp, salicylic acid is useful. It can be prescribed as 2-5% in aqueous cream, 1-2% in arachis oil, or 6% gel.

It is often easiest for the patient to apply the preparation to the scalp at night and wash it out the next morning with a tar shampoo.

Infection

Remember that secondary infection is a cause of persisting lesions.

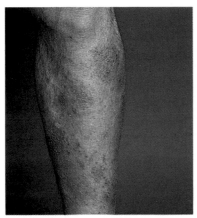
Lichenified eczema.

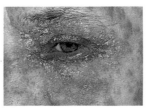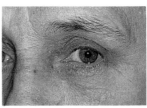
Infected eczema. Before and after treatment.

Hand dermatitis

<table>
<tr><td>

Hand dermatitis: hints on management

(1) Hand washing:
Use tepid water and soap without perfume or colouring or chemicals added. Dry carefully, especially between fingers.

(2) When in wet work:
Wear cotton gloves under rubber gloves (or plastic if you are allergic to rubber). Try not to use hot water and cut down to 15 minutes at a time if possible. Remove rings before wet or dry work. Use running water if possible.

(3) Wear gloves in cold weather and for dusty work.

(4) Use only ointments prescribed for you.

(5) Things to avoid:
  (a) Shampoo
  (b) Peeling fruits and vegetables, especially citrus fruits
  (c) Polishes of all kinds
  (d) Solvents—eg, white spirit, thinners, turpentine
  (e) Hair lotions, creams, and dyes
  (f) Detergents and strong cleansing agents
  (g) "Unknown" chemicals.

(6) Use "moisturisers" or emollients which have been recommended by your doctor—to counteract dryness.

</td></tr>
</table>

Hand dermatitis poses a particular problem in management and it is important that protection is continued after the initial rash has healed since it takes some time for the skin to recover its barrier function. Ointments or creams should be reapplied each time the hands have been washed.

It is useful to give patients a list of simple instructions such as those shown here.

Management of pruritus (itching skin)

<table>
<tr><td>

Causes

Endocrine diseases—Diabetes, myxoedema, hyperthyroidism.
Metabolic diseases—Hepatic failure, chronic renal failure.
Malignancy—Lymphoma, reticulosis, carcinomatosis.
Psychological—Anxiety, parasitophobia.
Tropical Infection—Filariasis, hookworm.
Drugs—Alkaloids.

</td></tr>
</table>

Scratching the skin produces lichenification so that it is not always possible to know if there was originally an underlying area of eczema or a primary itching condition of the skin.

Endogenous eczema can produce severe itching, often made worse by secondary infection. Irritants or allergens also cause an intense itching and should be suspected, particularly if the eyelids or hands are affected.

Scabies causes intense itching and can be overlooked. Take scrapings for mycological examination. In the absence of any other apparent condition remember the causes of pruritus shown in the box.

Treatment—The object of symptomatic treatment is to break the "itch-scratch-itch" cycle once the cause has been eliminated. Topical steroid ointments and occlusive dressings help to prevent scratching.

Treatment of eczema and inflammatory dermatoses

Use emollients for dry skin.

Topical local anaesthetics give relief but can cause allergic reactions. Sedative antihistamines at night may be helpful.

In liver failure cholestyramine powders may help to relieve the intense pruritus that can occur.

Pruritus ani is a common, troublesome condition and the following points may be helpful.

(1) Patients often wash obsessively and attack the perianal area frequently with soap and water. Advise gentle cleaning, once daily.

(2) Avoid harsh toilet paper—especially if it is coloured (cheap dyes irritate and can cause allergies). Olive oil and cotton wool can be used instead.

(3) Weaker topical steroids can be used to reduce inflammation with zinc cream or ointment as a protective layer on top.

(4) Anal leakage from an incompetent sphincter, skin tags, or haemorrhoids may require surgical treatment.

(5) There may be anxiety or depression but pruritus ani itself can lead to irritability and depression.

RASHES WITH EPIDERMAL CHANGES

| Lichen planus |
| Seborrhoeic dermatitis |
| Pityriasis rosea |
| Pityriasis lichenoides |
| Localised lesions |

Familiarity with the clinical features of psoriasis and eczema, which all clinicians see from time to time, provides a basis for comparison with other rather less common conditions.

The characteristics that each condition has in common with psoriasis and eczema are highlighted.

Lichen planus

Clinical features of psoriasis	*Clinical features of eczema*
Possible family history	Possible family history
Sometimes related to stress	Sometimes worse with stress
Itching—rare	Usually itching
Extensor surfaces and trunk	Flexor surfaces and face
Well defined, raised lesions	Poorly demarcated lesions
Hyperkeratosis	Oedema, vesicles, lichenification
Scaling, bleeding points beneath scales	Secondary infection sometimes present
Köbner phenomenon	
Nails affected	
Scalp affected	
Mucous membranes not affected	

Like psoriasis, the lesions are well defined and raised. They also occur in areas of trauma—the Köbner phenomenon. *Unlike* psoriasis, there is no family history and no particular relation to stress. Itching is common. The distribution is on the flexor aspects of the limbs, particularly the ankles and wrists, rather than on the extensor surfaces, as in psoriasis. However, a localised form of lichen planus occurs on the shin.

The typical flat topped lesions have a shiny hyperkeratotic lichenified surface with a violaceous colour, interrupted by milky white streaks—Wickham's striae. The oral mucosa is commonly affected with a white, net like appearance and sometimes ulceration.

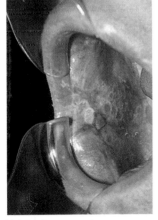

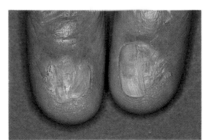

Lichen planus—nail.

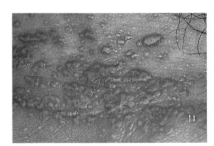

Lichen planus—skin.

Lichen planus—oral mucosa.

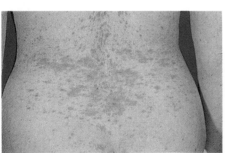

Lichen planus.

Less commonly very thick hypertrophic lesions occur and also follicular lesions. Lichen planus is one cause of localised alopecia on the scalp as a result of hair follicle destruction.

Nail disease is less common than in psoriasis. There may be thinning and atrophy of part or all of a nail and these often take the form of a longitudinal groove.

Lichen planus usually resolves over many months to leave residual brown or grey macules. In the oral mucosa and areas subject to trauma ulceration can occur.

Rashes with epidermal changes

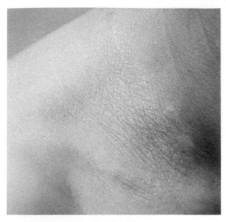

Lichenified eczema.

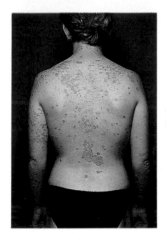

Guttate psoriasis.

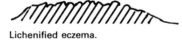

Lichenified eczema.

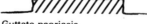

Guttate psoriasis.

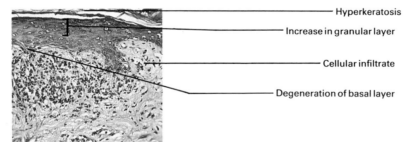

Hyperkeratosis
Increase in granular layer
Cellular infiltrate
Degeneration of basal layer

Similar rashes

Lichenified eczema—This is also itchy and may occur on the ankles and wrists. The edge of the lesion is less well defined and is irregular. The flat topped, shiny papules are absent.

Guttate psoriasis is not as itchy as lichen planus. Scaling erythematous lesions do not have the lichenified surface of lichen planus.

Pityriasis lichenoides—The lesions have a mica like scale overlying an erythematous papule.

Drug eruptions—Rashes with many features of lichen planus can occur in patients taking:

> Chloroquine
> Chlorpropamide } The 3 "C"s
> Chlorothiazide
> Anti-inflammatory drugs
> Gold preparations

It also occurs in those handling colour developers.

Treatment

The main symptom of itching is relieved to some extent by moderately potent steroid ointments. Very hypertrophic lesions may respond to strong steroid preparations under polythene occlusion. I have found careful intralesional injections very effective in persistent lesions. In very extensive, severe lichen planus systemic steroids may be indicated.

Lichen planus

Flexor surfaces
Mucous membranes affected
Itching common
Violaceous colour
Wickham's striae
Small discrete lesions
Lichenified

Pathology of lichen planus

As expected, there is hypertrophy and thickening of the epidermis with increased keratin. The white streaks seen clinically occur where there is pronounced thickness of the granular layer and underlying infiltrate. Degenerating basal cells may form "colloid bodies." The basal layer is being eaten away by an aggressive band of lymphocytes, the remaining papillae having a "saw toothed" appearance.

Seborrhoeic dermatitis

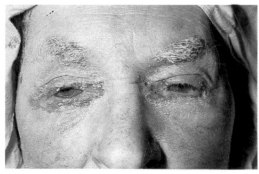

Seborrhoeic dermatitis.

Seborrhoeic dermatitis has nothing to do with sebum or any other kind of greasiness. There are two distinct types, adult and infantile.

Adult seborrhoeic dermatitis

The adult type is more common in men and in those with a tendency to scaling and dandruff in the scalp. There are several commonly affected areas.

(*a*) Seborrhoeic dermatitis affects the central part of the face, scalp, ears, and eyebrows. There may be an associated blepharitis, giving some red eyes and also otitis externa.

(*b*) The lesions over the sternum sometimes start as a single "medallion" lesion. A flower like "petaloid" pattern can occur. The back may be affected as well.

(*c*) Lesions also occur in well defined areas in the axillae and groin and beneath the breasts.

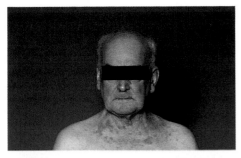

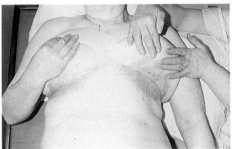

Seborrhoeic dermatitis.

Typically the lesions are discrete and erythematous and they may develop a yellow crust. The lesions tend to develop from the hair follicles. It is a persistent condition that varies in severity.

Clinically and pathologically the condition has features of both psoriasis and eczema. There is thickening of the epidermis with some of the inflammatory changes of psoriasis and the intercellular oedema of eczema. Parakeratosis—the presence of nuclei above the basement layer—may be noticeable. In recent years an increased number of *Pityrasporum ovale*, a normal commensal yeast, have been found.

Treatment—Topical steroids produce a rapid improvement, but not permanent clearing. Topical preparations containing salicylic acid, sulphur, or ichthammol may help in long term control. Ketoconazole by mouth has been reported to produce clearing and can be used topically. These drugs clear yeasts and fungi from the skin, including *P ovale*, which is further evidence for the role of this organism.

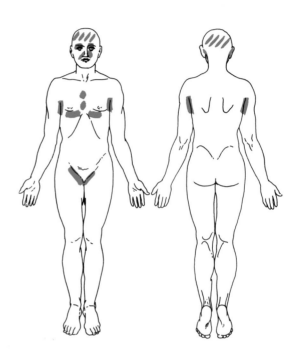

Clinical features of psoriasis	Clinical features of eczema
Possible family history	Possible family history
Sometimes related to stress	Sometimes worse with stress
Itching—rare	Usually itching
Extensor surfaces and trunk	Flexor surfaces and face
Well defined, raised lesions	Poorly demarcated lesions
Hyperkeratosis	Oedema, vesicles, lichenification
Scaling, bleeding points beneath scales	Secondary infection sometimes present
Köbner phenomenon	
Nails affected	
Scalp affected	
Mucous membranes not affected	

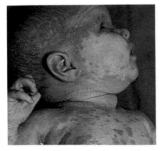

Infantile seborrhoeic dermatitis.

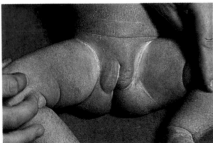

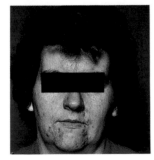

Perioral dermatitis.

Infantile seborrhoeic dermatitis

In young infants a florid red eruption occurs with well defined lesions on the trunk and confluent areas in the flexures associated with scaling of the scalp. There is no consistent association with the adult type of seborrhoeic dermatitis. It has been suggested that infantile seborrhoeic dermatitis is a variant of atopic eczema. A high proportion of affected infants develop atopic eczema later but there are distinct differences.

Itching is present in atopic eczema but not in seborrhoeic dermatitis.

The clinical course of atopic eczema is prolonged with frequent exacerbations, whereas seborrhoeic dermatitis clears in a few weeks and seldom recurs.

Allergy—IgE concentrations are often raised in atopic eczema and food allergy is frequent, but not in seborrhoeic dermatitis.

Perioral dermatitis

Perioral dermatitis is possibly a variant of seborrhoeic dermatitis, with some features of acne. Papules and pustules develop around the mouth and chin. It occurs mainly in women.

Rashes with epidermal changes
Pityriasis rosea

Lichen planus
Seborrhoeic dermatitis
Pityriasis rosea
Pityriasis lichenoides
Localised lesions

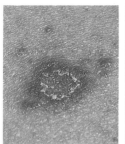 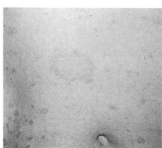 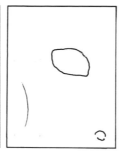

Herald lesions.

The word "pityriasis" is from the Greek for bran, and the fine bran like scales on the surface are a characteristic feature. The numerous pale pink oval or round patches can be confused with psoriasis or discoid eczema. The history helps since this condition develops as an acute eruption and the patient can often point to a simple initial lesion—the herald patch.

There is commonly slight itching. Pityriasis rosea occurs mainly in the second and third decade, often during the winter months. "Clusters" of cases occur but not true epidemics. This suggests an infective basis. There may be prodromal symptoms with malaise, fever, or lymphadenopathy. Numerous causes have been suggested from allergy to fungi; the current favourite is a virus infection.

The typical patient is an adolescent or young adult, who is often more than a little concerned about the sudden appearance of a widespread rash. The lesions are widely distributed, often following skin creases, and concentrated on the trunk with scattered lesions on the limbs. The face and scalp may be affected.

Early lesions are red with fine scales—usually 1-4 cm in diameter. The initial herald patch is larger and may be confused with a fungal infection. Subsequently the widespread eruption develops in a matter of days or, rarely, weeks. As time goes by the lesions clear to give a grey pigmentation with a collarette of scales facing towards the centre.

Clinical features of psoriasis	Clinical features of eczema
Possible family history	Possible family history
Sometimes related to stress	Sometimes worse with stress
Itching—rare	Usually itching
Extensor surfaces and trunk	Flexor surfaces and face
Well defined, raised lesions	Poorly demarcated lesions
Hyperkeratosis	Oedema, vesicles, lichenification
Scaling, bleeding points beneath scales	Secondary infection sometimes present
Köbner phenomenon	
Nails affected	
Scalp affected	
Mucous membranes not affected	

Similar rashes

Discoid eczema presents with itching and lesions with erythema, oedema, and crusting rather than scaling. Vesicles may be present. The rash persists unchanged.

A *drug eruption* can sometimes produce similar lesions.

Guttate psoriasis—The lesions are more sharply defined and smaller (0·5-1·0 cm) and have waxy scales.

The pathology of pityriasis rosea

Histological changes are non-specific, showing slight inflammatory changes in the dermis, oedema, and slight hyperkeratosis.

Pityriasis lichenoides

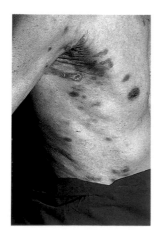

Pityriasis lichenoides is a less common condition occurring in acute and chronic forms.

The *acute* form presents with widespread pink papules which itch and form crusts, sometimes with vesicle formation suggestive of chickenpox. There may be ulceration. The lesions may develop in crops and resolve over a matter of weeks.

The *chronic* form presents as reddish brown papules—often with a "mica" like scale that reveals a smooth, red surface underneath, unlike the bleeding points of psoriasis. In lichen planus there is no superficial scale and blistering is unusual.

The distribution is over the trunk, thighs, and arms, usually sparing the face and scalp.

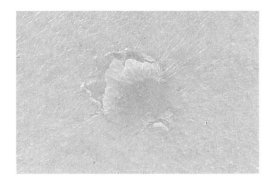

The underlying pathology—vascular dilatation and a lymphocytic infiltrate with a keratotic scale—is in keeping with the clinical appearance. The cause is unknown. Treatment is with topical steroids.

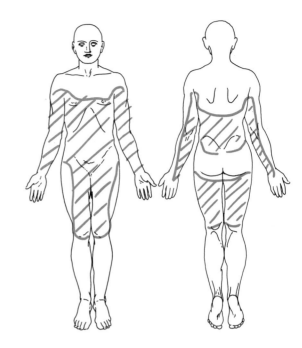

Clinical features of psoriasis	Clinical features of eczema
Possible family history	Possible family history
Sometimes related to stress	Sometimes worse with stress
Itching—rare	Usually itching
Extensor surfaces and trunk	Flexor surfaces and face
Well defined, raised lesions	Poorly demarcated lesions
Hyperkeratosis	Oedema, vesicles, lichenification
Scaling, bleeding points beneath scales	Secondary infection sometimes present
Köbner phenomenon	
Nails affected	
Scalp affected	
Mucous membranes not affected	

Pityriasis versicolor

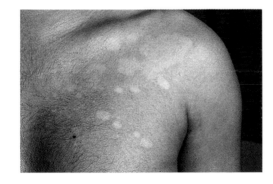

Pityriasis versicolor is a skin eruption that usually develops after sun exposure with white macules on the tanned skin but pale brown patches on the covered areas—hence the name—versicolor, or variable colour. The lesions are: (a) flat; (b) only *partially* depigmented—areas of vitiligo are totally white; and (c) do not show inflammation or vesicles.

The causative organism is a yeast—*Pityrosporum orbiculare*—that takes advantage of some unknown change in the epidermis and develops a proliferative, stubby, mycelial form—called malassezia furfur. This otherwise incidental information can be simply put to practical use by taking a superficial scraping from a lesion on to a microscope slide—add a drop of potassium hydroxide or water with a coverslip. The organisms are readily seen under the microscope: spherical yeast forms and mycelial rods, resembling "grapes and bananas" ("spaghetti and meatballs" in the United States).

Treatment is simple: selenium sulphide shampoo applied regularly with ample water while showering or bathing will clear the infection. The colour change may take some time to clear. Expensive antifungal preparations are not usually needed.

Desquamating stage of generalised erythema

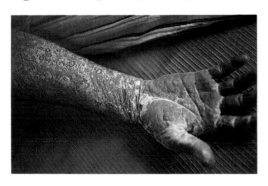

Any extensive acute erythema, from the erythroderma of psoriasis to a penicillin rash, commonly shows a stage of shedding large flakes of skin—desquamation—as it resolves. If only this stage is seen it can be confused with psoriasis.

Localised lesions with epidermal changes

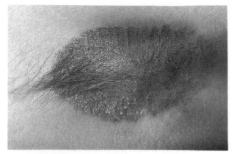

Flexural seborrhoeic dermatitis.

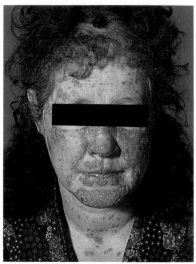

Systemic lupus erythematosus.

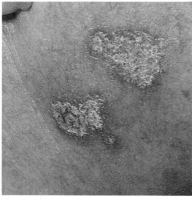

Discoid lupus erythematosus.

Psoriasis, seborrhoeic dermatitis, atopic eczema, and contact dermatitis can all present with localised lesions.

Psoriasis may affect only the flexures, occur as genital lesion, or affect only the palms. The lack of itching and epidermal changes with a sharp edge help in differentiation from infective or infiltrative lesions.

Seborrhoeic dermatitis can occur in the axillae or scalp with no lesions of other areas.

Atopic eczema—The "classical" sites in children—flexures of the elbows and knees and the face—may be modified to localised vesicular lesions on the hands and feet in older patients. Some atopic adults develop severe, persistent generalised eczematous changes.

Contact dermatitis is usually localised, by definition, to the areas in contact with irritant or allergen. Wide areas can be affected in reactions to clothing or washing powder, and sometimes the reaction extends beyond the site of contact.

Fungal infections—Apart from athlete's foot, toenail infections, and tinea cruris (in men) "ringworm" is in fact not nearly as common as is supposed. The damp, soggy, itching skin of athlete's foot is well known. An itching, red diffuse rash in the groin differentiates tinea cruris from psoriasis. However, a bacterial infection, erythrasma, may be confused with seborrhoeic dermatitis and psoriasis—skin scrapings can be taken for culture of *Corynebacterium minutissimum* or, more simply, green/blue fluorescence shown with Wood's light. The scaling macules from dog and cat ringworm (*Microsporum canis*) itch greatly while the indurated pustular, boggy lesion (kerion) of the cattle ringworm is quite distinctive.

Fungal infection of the axillae is rare; a red rash here is more likely to be due to erythrasma or seborrhoeic dermatitis.

Tinea cruris is very unusual before puberty and is uncommon in women.

In all cases of suspected fungal infection skin scrapings should be taken on to black paper, in which they can be folded and sent to the laboratory. In some units special "kits" are provided, which contain folded black paper and Sellotape strips on slides for taking a superficial layer of epidermis.

Lupus erythematosus—There are two forms of this condition: *discoid*, which is generally limited to the skin, and *systemic*, in which the skin changes are associated with disease of the kidneys and other organs. The acute, erythematous rash on the malar area of the face, usually in a woman, is characteristic of the systemic type. In discoid lupus erythematosus there are well defined lesions, which are a combination of atrophy and hyperkeratosis of the follicles, giving a "nutmeg grater" feel. It occurs predominantly on the face or areas exposed to the sun as chronic, erythematous lesions that are much worse in the summer months.

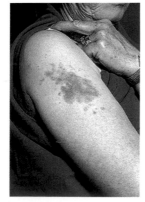

Fixed drug eruption.

Fixed drug eruptions—Generalised drug eruptions are considered under erythema, but there is a localised form recurring every time the drug is used. There is usually a well defined, erythematous plaque, sometimes with vesicles. Crusting, scaling, and pigmentation occur as the lesion heals. It is usually found on the limbs, and more than one lesion can occur.

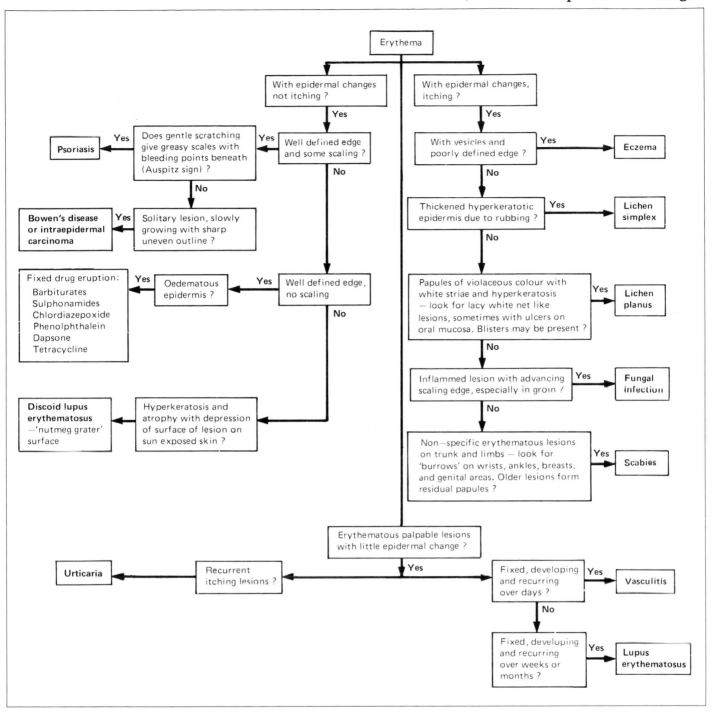

Erythema

With epidermal changes not itching ? → **Yes**

With epidermal changes, itching ? → **Yes**

Yes → Does gentle scratching give greasy scales with bleeding points beneath (Auspitz sign) ? → **Yes** → Well defined edge and some scaling ?

Yes → Psoriasis

No (from Auspitz) → Solitary lesion, slowly growing with sharp uneven outline ? → **Yes** → **Bowen's disease or intraepidermal carcinoma**

Well defined edge and some scaling ? → **No**

With vesicles and poorly defined edge ? → **Yes** → Eczema
No → Thickened hyperkeratotic epidermis due to rubbing ? → **Yes** → **Lichen simplex**
No → Papules of violaceous colour with white striae and hyperkeratosis — look for lacy white net like lesions, sometimes with ulcers on oral mucosa. Blisters may be present ? → **Yes** → **Lichen planus**
No → Inflammed lesion with advancing scaling edge, especially in groin ? → **Yes** → **Fungal infection**
No → Non—specific erythematous lesions on trunk and limbs — look for 'burrows' on wrists, ankles, breasts, and genital areas. Older lesions form residual papules ? → **Yes** → Scabies

Fixed drug eruption:
  Barbiturates
  Sulphonamides
  Chlordiazepoxide
  Phenolphthalein
  Dapsone
  Tetracycline
← **Yes** — Oedematous epidermis ? ← **Yes** — Well defined edge, no scaling

Well defined edge, no scaling → **No**

Discoid lupus erythematosus —'nutmeg grater' surface ← Hyperkeratosis and atrophy with depression of surface of lesion on sun exposed skin ?

Erythematous palpable lesions with little epidermal change ? → **Yes**

Urticaria ← Recurrent itching lesions ? ← **Yes** — Fixed, developing and recurring over days ? → **Yes** → Vasculitis

Fixed, developing and recurring over days ? → **No** → Fixed, developing and recurring over weeks or months ? → **Yes** → Lupus erythematosus

25

RASHES ARISING IN THE DERMIS

The erythemas

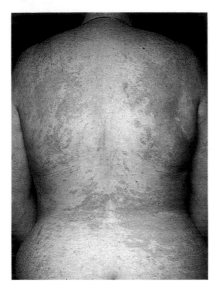

Erythema from antibiotics.

Causes of "toxic" erythema

Drugs	antibiotics, barbiturates, thiazides
Infections	any recent infection such as streptococcal throat infection or erysipelas; spirochaetal infections; viral infections
Pregnancy	
Systemic disease	lupus erythematosus

Complex reactions occurring in the capillaries and arterioles of the skin cause erythema—which is simply redness of the skin. This may present as flat macules or as papules, which are raised above the surrounding skin. The lesions may be transient or last for weeks, constant or variable in distribution, with or without vesicles.

It is possible to recognise specific patterns within this plethora of clinical signs, but even the most experienced dermatologist may be reduced to making a general diagnosis of "toxic" erythema. The best we can do therefore is to recognise the common types of erythema and list the possible causes. It is then a matter of deciding on the most likely underlying condition or group of conditions—for example, bacterial infection or autoimmune systemic disease.

Morphology and distribution

Because there can be the same cause for a variety of erythematous rashes detailed descriptions are of limited use. None the less, there are some characteristic patterns.

Morbilliform—The presentation of measles is well known, with the appearance of Koplik's spots on the mucosa, photophobia with conjunctivitis, and red macules behind the ears, spreading to the face, trunk, and limbs. The prodromal symptoms and conjunctivitis are absent in drug eruptions. Other viral conditions, including those caused by echoviruses, rubella, infectious mononucleosis, and erythema infectiosum may have to be considered.

Scarlatiniform rashes are similar to that in scarlet fever, when an acute erythematous eruption occurs in relation to a streptococcal infection. Characteristically erythema is widespread on the trunk. There is intense erythema and engorgement of the pharyngeal lymphoid tissue with an exudate and a "strawberry" tongue. Bacterial infections can produce a similar rash, as can drug rashes, without the systemic symptoms.

Erythema multiforme

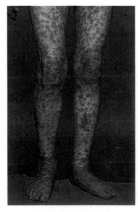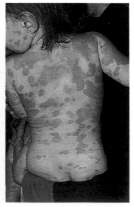

Erythema multiforme.

Erythema multiforme is sometimes misdiagnosed because of the variety of lesions and number of possible precipitating causes; some of these are listed below.

Infections	*Neoplasia*
Herpes simplex—the commonest cause	Hodgkin's disease
	Myeloma
Mycoplasma infection	Carcinoma
Infectious mononucleosis	*Chronic inflammation*
Poliomyelitis (vaccine)	Sarcoidosis
Many other viral and bacterial infections	Wegener's granuloma
	Drugs
Any focal sepsis	Barbiturates
BCG inoculation	Sulphonamides
Collagen disease	Penicillin
Systemic lupus erythematosus	Phenothiazine and many
Polyarteritis nodosa	others

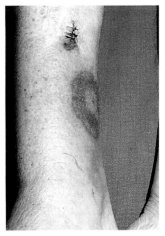

Annular lesions of erythema multiforme.

Clinical picture

The usual erythematous lesions occur in crops on the limbs and trunk. Each lesion may extend, leaving a cyanotic centre, which produces an "iris" or "target" lesion. Bullae may develop in the lesions and on the mucous membranes. A severe bullous form, with lesions on the mucous membranes, is known as the Stevens-Johnson syndrome. There may be neural and bronchial changes as well. Barbiturates, sulphonamides, and other drugs are the most common cause.

Histologically there are inflammatory changes, vasodilatation, and degeneration of the epidermis.

A condition that may be confused is *Sweet's syndrome*, which presents as acute plum coloured raised painful lesions on the limbs—sometimes the face and neck—with fever. It is more common in women. The alternative name, "acute febrile neutrophilic dermatosis," describes the presentation and the pathological findings of a florid neutrophilic infiltrate. There is often a preceding upper respiratory infection. Treatment with steroids produces a rapid response but recurrences are common.

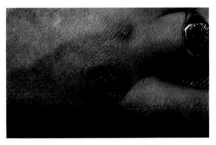

Annular lesions of erythema multiforme.

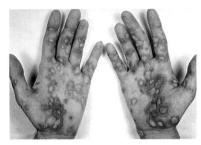

Blistering lesions.

Erythema induratum

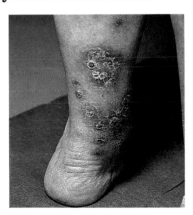

Erythema induratum occurs on the lower legs posteriorly, usually in women, with diffuse, indurated dusky red lesions that may ulcerate. It is more common in patients with poor cutaneous circulation. Epithelioid cell granulomas may form and at one time it was thought to be associated with tuberculosis.

In other patients recurrent erythematous nodules occur in the lower calf.

Erythema nodosum

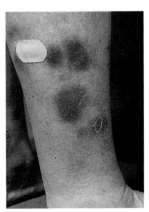

Erythema nodosum occurs as firm, gradually developing lesions, predominantly on the extensor aspect of the legs. They are tender and progress from an acute erythematous stage to residual lesions resembling bruises over four to eight weeks.

Usually multiple lesions occur varying in size from 1 to 5 cm. The lesions are usually preceded by an upper respiratory tract infection and may be associated with fever and arthralgia. Infections (streptococcal, tuberculous, viral, and fungal) and sarcoidosis are the commonest underlying conditions. Drugs, too, can precipitate erythema nodosum, the contraceptive pill and the sulphonamides being the commonest cause. Ulcerative colitis and lymphoma may also be associated with the condition.

Rashes arising in the dermis
Rashes due to drugs

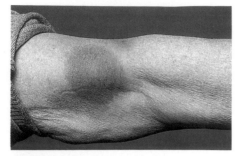

Fixed drug eruption.

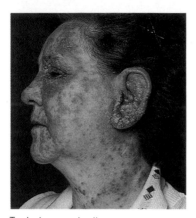

Topical neomycin allergy.

There is an almost infinite variety of types of drug reaction. The more usual clinical presentations provide a basic framework with which variations can be compared.

External contact with drugs can cause a contact dermatitis presenting with eczematous changes. This occurs commonly with neomycin and bacitracin. Chloramphenicol and sulphonamides from ophthalmic preparations can also cause dermatitis around the eyes. Penicillin is a potent sensitiser so is not used for topical treatment.

Drugs used *systemically* can cause a localised fixed drug eruption or a more diffuse macular or papular erythema, symmetrically distributed. In the later stages exfoliation, with shedding scales of skin, may develop. Antibiotics, particularly penicillins, are the most common cause. They also cause erythema multiforme as already mentioned.

Penicillins are the most common cause of drug rashes, which range from acute anaphylaxis to persistent diffuse erythematous lesions. Joint pains, fever, and proteinuria may be associated, as in serum sickness.

Ampicillin often produces a characteristic erythematous maculopapular rash on the limbs 7-20 days after the start of treatment. Such rashes occur in nearly all patients with infectious mononucleosis who are given ampicillin.

Other reactions

Blistering eruptions—Barbiturates	*Lichen planus-*	
Sulphonamides	*like reactions* —Chloroquine	
Iodines/		Chlorothiazide
bromides		Chlorpropamide
Chlorpropamide	*Photosensitivity* —Thiazide diuretics	
Salicylates	(seen on areas	Sulphonamides
Phenylbutazone	exposed to	Tetracyclines
	light)	

Vasculitis

Vasculitis

Inflammation around dilated capillaries and small blood vessels:

● a common component of the erythemas
● may occur as red macules and papules with necrotic lesions on the extremities
● in children a purpuric type (Henoch-Schönlein purpura) occurs in association with nephritis
● systemic lesions may occur, with renal, joint, gastrointestinal, and central nervous system involvement.

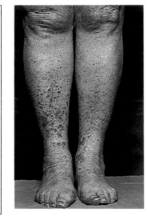

Inflammation associated with capillary and small blood vessels is part of the pathological changes of many of the conditions described above. The term vasculitis is also used clinically to describe a variable clinical picture with red macules and papules and with necrosis and bruising in severe cases. In children purpura is more prominent and these cases are classified as Henoch-Schönlein purpura. The legs and arms are usually affected. Skin signs are preceded by malaise and fever with arthropathy and there may be associated urticaria. Since a high proportion of cases are associated with systemic lesions it is essential to check for renal, joint, gastrointestinal, and central nervous system disease. In children with Henoch-Schönlein purpura nephritis is common.

Purpura

Is seen on the skin as a result of:

● thrombocytopenia—platelet deficiency
● senile purpura—due to shearing of capillaries as a result of defective supporting connective tissue
● purpura in patients on corticosteroid treatment—similar to senile purpura
● Schamberg's disease—brown macules and red spots resembling cayenne pepper on the legs of men
● associated vasculitis.

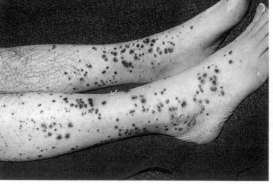

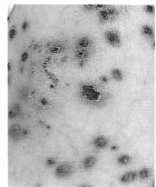

Acute vasculitis with necrosis.

Urticaria

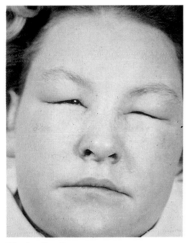

Urticaria.

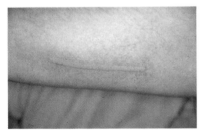

Giant urticaria.

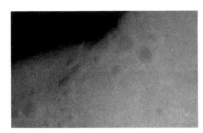

Dermatographism.

In this condition itching red weals develop; they resemble the effects of stinging nettle (*Urtica Dioica*) on the skin. The condition may be associated with allergic reactions, infection, or physical stimuli, but in most patients no cause can be found. Similar lesions may precede, or be associated with, vasculitis (*urticarial vasculitis*), pemphigoid, or dermatitis herpetiformis.

The histological changes may be very slight but usually there is oedema, vasodilation, and a cellular infiltrate of lymphocytes, polymorphs, and histiocytes. Various vasoactive substances are thought to be involved, including histamine, kinins, leukotrines, prostaglandins, and complement.

Angio-oedema is due to oedema of the subcutaneous tissues; it can occur rapidly and may involve the mucous membranes. *Hereditary angio-oedema* is a rare form with recurrent severe episodes of subcutaneous oedema, swelling of the mucous membranes, and systemic symptoms. Laryngeal oedema is the most serious complication.

The physical urticarias, which account for about 25% of cases, include *dermatographism* and the *pressure, cold, heat, solar, cholinergic*, and *aquagenic urticarias*.

Dermatographism is an exaggerated response to stroking the skin firmly with a hard object, such as the end of a pencil. *Pressure urticaria* is caused by sustained pressure from clothing, hard seats, and footwear; it may last some hours. *Cold urticaria* varies in severity and is induced by cold, particularly by cold winds or by the severe shock of bathing in cold water. It appears early in life—in infancy in the rare familial form. In a few cases abnormal serum proteins may be found. *Heat urticaria* is rare, but warm environments often make physical urticaria worse. *Solar urticaria* is a rare condition in which sunlight causes an acute urticarial eruption. Tolerance to sun exposure may develop in areas of the body normally exposed to sun. There is sensitivity to a wide spectrum of ultraviolet light. *Cholinergic urticaria* is characterised by the onset of itching urticarial papules after exertion, stress, or exposure to heat. The injection of cholinergic drugs induces similar lesions in some patients. *Aquagenic urticaria* occurs on contact with water, regardless of the temperature.

Non-physical urticaria may be *acute* in association with allergic reactions to insect bites, drugs, and other factors. Chronic recurrent urticaria is fairly common. Innumerable causes have been suggested but, to the frustration of patient and doctor alike, it is often impossible to identify any specific factor. Some reported causes are listed below.

BLISTERS AND PUSTULES

Development, duration, and distribution

<table>
<tr><td colspan="3">

The differential diagnosis of blistering eruptions

Widespread blisters

Eczema—Lichenification and crusting, itching

Dermatitis herpetiformis—Itching, extensor surface, persistent

Chickenpox—Crops of blisters, self limiting, prodromal illness

Pityriasis lichenoides—pink papules, developing blisters

Erythema multiforme—erythematous and "target" lesions, mucous membranes affected

Pemphigoid—Older patients, trunk and flexures affected. Preceding erythematous lesions, deeply situated, tense blisters

Pemphigus—Adults, widespread superficial blisters, mucous membranes affected (erosions)

Drug eruptions—History of drugs prescribed, overdose (barbiturates, tranquillisers)

Localised blisters

Eczema—"Pompholyx" blisters on hands and feet, itching

Allergic reactions, including topical medication, insect bites

Psoriasis—Deep, sterile, non-itching blisters on palms and soles

Impetigo—Usually localised, staphylococci and streptococci isolated

Herpes simplex—Itching lesions developing turbid blisters

</td></tr>
</table>

Several diseases may present with blisters or pustules. There is no common condition that can be used as a "reference point" with which less usual lesions can be compared as rashes can be compared with psoriasis. A different approach is needed for the assessment of blistering or pustular lesions, based on the history and appearance and summarised as the three Ds: development, duration, and distribution.

Development—Was there any preceding systemic illness—as in chickenpox, hand, foot, and mouth disease, and other viral infections? Was there a preceding area of erythema—as in herpes simplex or phemphigoid? Is the appearance of the lesions associated with itching—as in herpes simplex, dermatitis herpetiformis, and eczematous vesicles on the hands and feet?

Duration—Some acute blistering arises rapidly— for example, in allergic reactions, impetigo, erythema multiforme, and pemphigus. Other blisters have a more gradual onset and follow a chronic course—as in dermatitis herpetiformis, pityriasis lichenoides, and the bullae of porphyria cutanea tarda. The rare genetic disorder epidemolysis bullosa is present from, or soon after, birth.

Distribution—The distribution of blistering rashes helps considerably in making a clinical diagnosis. The most common patterns of those that have a fairly constant distribution are shown.

Itching is a very useful symptom. If all the accessible lesions are scratched and it is hard to find an intact blister it is probably an itching rash.

Itching	Non-itching	
Eczema-pompholyx on hands and feet	Erythema multiforme	Pustular psoriasis of hands and feet
Allergic reactions	Pemphigus vulgaris	
Dermatitis herpetiformis	Bullous pemphigoid	
Chickenpox	Bullous impetigo	
Herpes simplex	Insect bite allergy	

Clinical features: widespread blisters

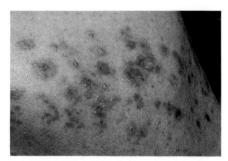

Dermatitis herpetiformis.

Chickenpox

Chickenpox is so well known in general practice that it is rarely seen in hospital clinics and is sometimes not recognised. The prodromal illness lasts one to two days and is followed by erythematous lesions that rapidly develop vesicles, then pustules, followed by crusts in two to three days. Crops of lesions develop at the same sites—usually on the trunk, face, scalp, and limbs. The oral mucosa may be affected. The condition is usually benign.

Dermatitis herpetiformis

Dermatitis herpetiformis occurs in early and middle adult life and is characterised by symmetrical, intensely itching vesicles on the trunk and extensor surfaces. The vesicles are superficial. The onset is gradual, but may occur rapidly. The distribution is shown in the diagram on the next page.

Blisters and pustules

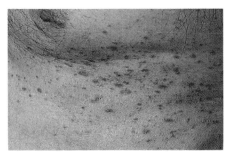

Dermatitis herpetiformis.

Variants of dermatitis herpetiformis are larger blisters forming bullae and erythematous papules and vesicles.

Associated conditions—Coeliac disease with villous atrophy and gluten intolerance may occur in association with dermatitis herpetiformis. Linear IgA disease is a more severe, widespread disease, in which there are "linear" deposits of IgA along the basement membrane of the epidermis and not only at the tips of the papillae as in dermatitis herpetiformis. Treatment is with Dapsone or sulphapyridine together with a gluten free diet.

Erythema multiforme with blisters

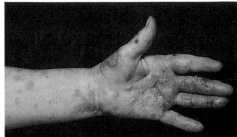

Erythema multiforme.

Blistering can occur on the lesions of erythema multiforme to a variable degree; when severe, generalised, and affecting the mucous membranes it is known as Stevens Johnson syndrome. The typical erythematous maculopapular changes develop over one to two days with a large blister (bulla) developing in the centre of the target lesions. In severe progressive cases there is extensive disease of the mouth, eyes, genitalia, and respiratory tract. The blisters are subepidermal— that is, deep—although some basement membrane remains on the floor of the blister.

Pityriasis lichenoides.

Pityriasis lichenoides varioliformis acuta

As the name implies, lichenified papules are the main feature of pityriasis lichenoides varioliformis acuta (or Mucha-Habermann's disease), but vesicles occur in the acute form. Crops of pink papules develop centrally, with vesicles, necrosis, and scales resembling those of chickenpox, hence the "varioliformis." There is considerable variation in the clinical picture, and a prodromal illness may occur. The condition may last from six weeks to six months. No infective agent has been isolated. The pathological changes parallel the clinical appearance with inflammation around the blood vessels and oedema within the dermis.

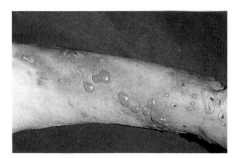

Bullous pemphigoid.

Pemphigoid

The bullous type of pemphigoid is a disease of the elderly in which tense bullae develop rapidly, often over a preceding erythematous rash, as well as on normal skin. The flexural aspects of the limbs and trunk are mainly affected. The bullae are subepidermal and persistent, with antibodies deposited at the dermoepidermal junction. Unlike pemphigus, there is a tendency for the condition to remit after many months. Treatment is with corticosteroids by mouth, 40 to 60 mg daily in most patients, although higher doses are required by some. Azathioprine aids remission, with reduced steroid requirements, but takes some weeks to produce an effect. Topical steroids can be used on developing lesions.

Chronic scarring pemphigoid affects the mucous membranes with small bullae that break down, leading to erosions and adhesions in the conjunctivae, mouth, pharynx, and genitalia.

There is also a localised type of pemphigoid occurring on the legs of elderly women that runs a benign self limiting course.

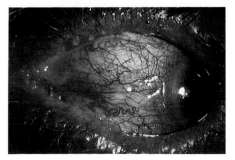

Mucous membrane pemphigoid.

Blisters and pustules

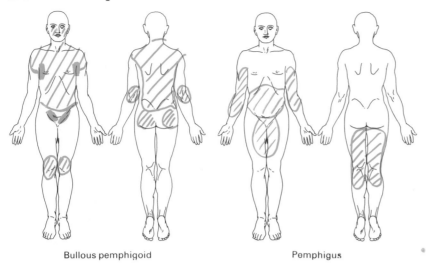

Bullous pemphigoid   Pemphigus

Pemphigus

The most common form of pemphigus vulgaris is a chronic progressive condition with widespread superficial bullae arising in normal skin. In about half of the cases this is preceded by blisters and erosions in the mouth. The bullae are easily broken, and even rubbing apparently normal skin causes the superficial epidermis to slough off (Nikolsky sign). These changes are associated with the deposition of immunoglobulin in the epidermal intercellular spaces. It is a serious condition with high morbidity despite treatment with steroids and azathioprine.

Pemphigus vegetans and pemphigus erythematosus are less common variants.

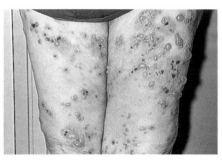

Pemphigus vulgaris.

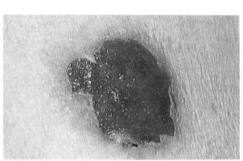

Nikolsky sign.

Ulcers in the mouth

Differential diagnosis:

Trauma (dentures)

Aphthous ulcers

Candida albicans infection

Herpes simplex

Erythema multiforme (from drugs)

Pemphigus

Lichen planus

Carcinoma

Clinical features: localised blisters

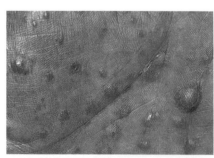

Pompholyx—which means "a bubble"—is characterised by persistent, itchy, clear blisters on the fingers, which may extend to the palms, with larger blisters. The feet may be affected. Secondary infection leads to turbid vesicle fluid. Pompholyx may be associated with a number of conditions— atopy, stress, fungal infection elsewhere, and allergic reactions. It may occur as a result of ingesting nickel in nickel sensitive patients and a similar reaction has been reported to neomycin.

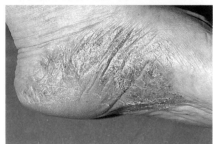

Pustular psoriasis is characterised by deep seated sterile blisters, often with no sign of psoriasis elsewhere— hence the term *palmopustular pustulosis*. Foci of sepsis have long been considered a causative factor and recent studies have shown a definite association with cigarette smoking. The pattern of HLA antigens indicates that this may be a separate condition from psoriasis.

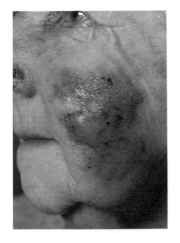

Bullous impetigo is seen in children and adults. Staphylococci are usually isolated from the blister fluid. The blisters are commonly seen on the face and are more deeply situated than in the non-bullous variety.

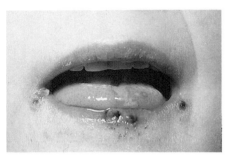
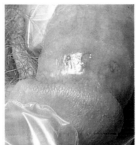

Herpes simplex—Primary infection with type I virus occurs on the face, lips, and buccal mucosa in children and young adults. Type II viruses cause genital infection. Itching may be severe.

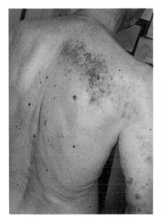
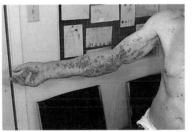

Herpes zoster is due to varicella virus producing groups of vesicles in a dermatome distribution, usually thoracic, trigeminal, or lumbosacral. It is more common after the fourth decade of life.

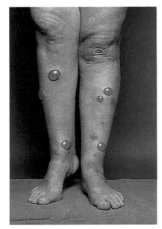
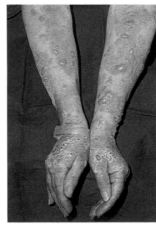

Insect bite allergy.   Drug reaction to sulphapyridine.

Insect bite allergy—Large blisters, which are usually not itching, can occur on the legs of susceptible individuals.

Bullous drug eruptions

Fixed drug eruptions can develop bullae, and some drugs can cause a generalised bullous eruption, particularly:

> Barbiturates (particularly if taken in overdosage)
> Sulphonamides
> Penicillamine (captopril, penicillins (which produce pemphigus-like bullae))
> Frusemide (may be phototoxic)

Remember that there may be an associated erythematous eruption.

LEG ULCERS

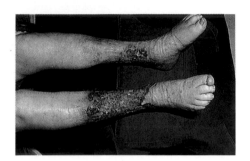

Although the patient will not probably die of this disease, yet, without great care, it may render her miserable. The disease may be very much relieved by art, and it is one of very common occurrence.

SIR BENJAMIN BRODIE (1846)

Despite the great increase in our understanding of the pathology of leg ulcers, their management is still largely "art." Consequently there are numerous treatments, each with their enthusiastic advocates. There are, however, basic concepts which are helpful in management. Since about 95% of leg ulcers are of the "venous" or gravitational variety these will be considered first.

Pathology of venous ulcers

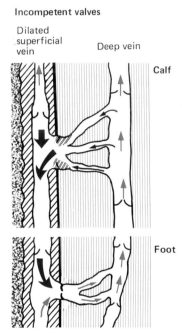

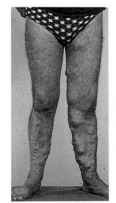

Varicose veins.

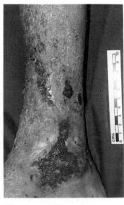

Ulcers and fibrosis.

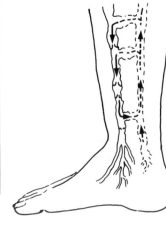

The skin—Ulcers arise because the skin dies from inadequate provision of nutrients and oxygen. This occurs as a consequence of (*a*) oedema in the subcutaneous tissues with poor lymphatic and capillary drainage; and (*b*) the extravascular accumulation of fibrinous material that has leaked from the blood vessels. The result is a rigid cuff around the capillaries, preventing diffusion through the wall, and fibrosis of the surrounding tissues.

The blood vessels—Arterial perfusion of the leg is usually normal or increased, but stasis occurs in the venules. The lack of venous drainage is a consequence of incompetent valves between the superficial veins and the deeper large veins on which the calf muscle "pump" acts. In the normal leg there is a *superficial* low pressure venous system and *deep* high pressure veins. If the blood flow from superficial to deep veins is reversed then the pressure in the superficial veins may increase to a level that prevents venous drainage with "back pressure" causing stasis and oedema.

Incompetent valves leading to gravitational ulcers may be preceded by:

(*a*) deep vein thrombosis associated with pregnancy or, less commonly, leg injury, immobilisation, or infarction in the past;

(*b*) primary long saphenous vein insufficiency;

(*c*) familial venous valve incompetence that presents at an earlier stage. There is a familial predisposition in half of all patients with leg ulcers; or

(*d*) deep venous obstruction.

Who gets ulcers?

Mainly women get ulcers—2% of those over 80 having venous ulcers as a long term consequence of the factors listed above. Leg ulcers are more likely to occur and are more severe in obese people.

Clinical changes

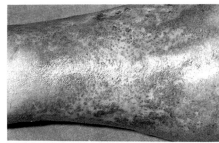

Atrophie blanche.

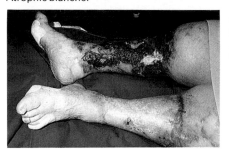

Champagne bottle legs.

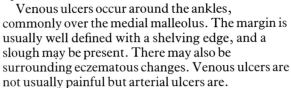

Oedema and fibrinous exudate often lead to fibrosis of the subcutaneous tissues, which may be associated with localised loss of pigment and dilated capillary loops, an appearance known as "atrophie blanche." This occurs around the ankle with oedema and dilated tortuous superficial veins proximally. This can lead to "champagne bottle legs," the bottle, of course, being inverted. Ulceration often occurs for the first time after a trivial injury.

Lymphoedema results from obliteration of the superficial lymphatics, with associated fibrosis. There is often hypertrophy of the overlying epidermis with a "polypoid" appearance, also known as lipodermatosclerosis.

Venous ulcers occur around the ankles, commonly over the medial malleolus. The margin is usually well defined with a shelving edge, and a slough may be present. There may also be surrounding eczematous changes. Venous ulcers are not usually painful but arterial ulcers are.

It is important to check the pulses in the leg and foot as compression bandaging of a leg with impaired blood flow can cause ischaemia and necrosis.

Treatment

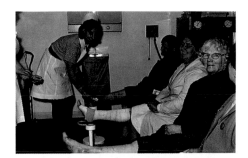

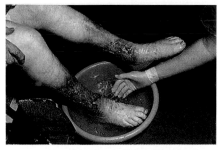

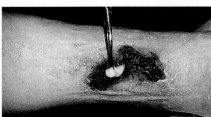

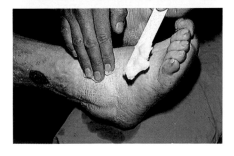

When new epidermis can grow across an ulcer it will and the aim is to produce an environment in which this can take place. To this end several measures can be taken.

(1) Oedema may be reduced by means of (a) diuretics, (b) keeping the legs elevated when sitting, (c) avoiding standing as far as possible. Raising the heels slightly from time to time helps venous return by the "calf muscle pump," (d) applying compression bandages, which may do more harm than good *unless* they are applied *before* the patient gets out of bed in the morning, when there is minimal oedema, and applied with more pressure on the foot than the calf, so as to create a pressure gradient towards the thigh.

(2) Exudate and slough should be removed. Lotions can be used to clean the ulcer and as compresses—0·9% saline solution, sodium hypochlorite solution, Eusol, or 5% hydrogen peroxide.

There is some evidence that antiseptic solutions and chlorinated solutions (such as sodium hypochlorite and Eusol) delay collagen production and cause inflammation. Enzyme preparations may help by "digesting" the slough. To prevent the formation of granulation tissue use silver nitrate 0·25% compresses, a silver nitrate "stick" for more exuberant tissue, and curettage, if necessary.

(3) The dressings applied to the ulcer can consist of (a) simple non-stick, paraffin gauze dressings. An allergy may develop to those with an antibiotic; (b) wet compresses with saline or silver nitrate solutions for exudative lesions; (c) silver sulphadiazine (Flamazine) or hydrogen peroxide creams (Hioxyl); and (d) absorbent dressings, consisting of hydrocolloid patches or powder, which are helpful for smaller ulcers.

(4) Paste bandages, impregnated with zinc oxide and antiseptics or ichthammol, help to keep dressings in place and provide protection. They may, however, traumatise the skin, and allergic reactions to their constituents are not uncommon.

(5) Treatment of infection is less often necessary than is commonly supposed. All ulcers are colonised by bacteria to some extent, usually coincidental staphylococci. A purulent exudate is an indication for a broad spectrum antibiotic and a swab for bacteriology. Erythema, oedema, and tenderness around the ulcer suggest a β haemolytic streptococcal infection, which will require long term antibiotic treatment. Dyes can be painted on

Systemic antibiotics have little effect on ulcers but are indicated if there is surrounding cellulitis. A swab for culture and sensitivity helps to keep track of organisms colonising the area.

Leg ulcers

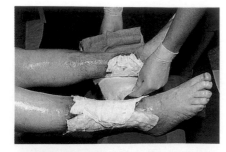

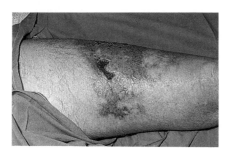

the edge of the ulcer, where they fix to the bacterial wall as well as the patient's skin. In Scotland bright red eosin is traditionally used, while in the south a blue dye, gentian violet, is favoured.

(6) Surrounding eczematous changes should be treated. Use topical steroids, not more than medium strength, avoiding the ulcer itself. Ichthammol 11% in 15% zinc oxide and white soft paraffin or Ichthopaste bandages can be used as a protective layer, and topical antibiotics can be used if necessary. It is important to remember that any of the commonly used topical preparations can cause an allergic reaction: neomycin, lanolin, formaldehyde, tars, Clinaform (the "C" of many proprietary steroids).

(7) Skin grafting can be very effective. There must be a healthy viable base for the graft, with an adequate blood supply; natural re-epithelialisation from the edges of the ulcer is a good indication that a graft will be supported. Pinch grafts or partial thickness grafts can be used. Any clinical infection, particularly with pseudomonal organisms, should be cleaned.

(8) Maintaining general health, with adequate nutrition and weight reduction, is important.

(9) Corrective surgery for associated venous abnormalities.

Arterial ulcers

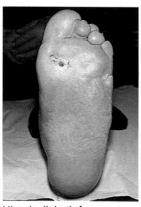

Ulcers on the leg also occur as a result of (a) atherosclerosis with poor peripheral circulation, particularly in older patients; (b) vasculitis affecting the larger subcutaneous arteries; and (c) arterial obstruction in macroglobulinaemia, cryoglobulinaemia, and polycythaemia "collagen" disease—particularly rheumatoid arthritis.

Arterial ulcers are sharply defined and accompanied by pain, which may be very severe, especially at night. The leg, especially the pretibial area, is affected rather than the ankle. In patients with hypertension a very tender ulcer can develop posteriorly (Martorelli's ulcer).

As mentioned above, compression bandaging will make arterial ulcers worse and may lead to ischaemia of the leg.

Diagnosis

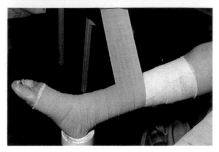

Ulcer in diabetic foot.

The differing presentation of arterial and venous ulcers helps in distinguishing between them, but some degree of arterial insufficiency often complicates venous ulcers.

Phlebography and Doppler ultrasound may help in detecting venous incompetence and arterial obstruction, which can sometimes be treated surgically.

Ulcers on the leg may also occur secondary to other diseases, because of infection, in malignant disease, and after trauma.

Secondary ulcers—Ulcers occur in diabetes, in periarteritis nodosa, and in vasculitis. Pyoderma gangrenosum, a chronic necrotic ulcer with surrounding induration, may occur in association with ulcerative colitis or rheumatoid vasculitis.

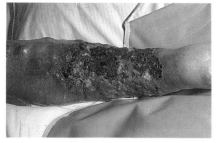

Squamous cell carcinoma in venous ulcer.

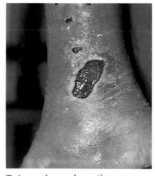

Tuberculous ulceration.

Infections that cause ulcers include staphylococcal or streptococcal infections, tuberculosis (which is rare in the United Kingdom but may be seen in recent immigrants), and anthrax.

Malignant diseases—Squamous cell carcinoma may present as an ulcer or, rarely, develop in a pre-existing ulcer. Basal cell carcinoma and melanoma may develop into ulcers, as may Kaposi's sarcoma.

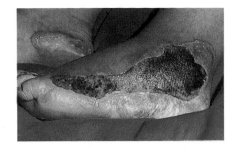

Trauma—Patients with diabetic or other types of neuropathy are at risk of developing trophic ulcers. Rarely they may be self induced—"dermatitis artefacta."

In treating venous leg ulcers
(1) Take measures to eliminate oedema and reduce weight—make sure the patient understands these.
(2) Never apply steroid preparations to the ulcer itself or it will not heal. Make sure that both nurses and patients are aware of this.
(3) Beware of allergy developing to topical agents—especially to antibiotics.

(4) There is no need to submit the patient to a variety of antibiotics according to the differing bacteria isolated from leg ulcers, unless there is definite evidence of infection clinically.
(5) A vascular "flare" round the ankle and heel with varicose veins, sclerosis, or oedema indicates a high risk of ulceration developing.
(6) Make sure arterial pulses are present.

ACNE AND ROSACEA

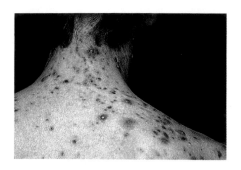

Acne goes with adolescence, a term derived from the Greek "acme" or prime of life. The young girl who is desperately aware of the smallest comedo and the otherwise handsome young man, with his face or back a battle field of acne cysts and scars, are familiar to us all.

What is acne?

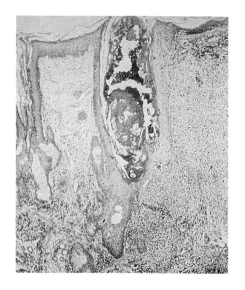

Acne lesions develop from the sebaceous glands associated with hair follicles—on the face, external auditory meatus, back, chest, and anogenital area. (Sebaceous glands are also found on the eyelids and mucosa, prepuce and cervix, where they are not associated with hair follicles.) The sebaceous gland contains holocrine cells that secrete triglycerides, fatty acids, wax esters, and sterols as "sebum." The main changes in acne are:

(*a*) an increase in sebum secretion;
(*b*) thickening of the keratin lining of the sebaceous duct, to produce blackheads or comedones. The colour of blackheads is due to melanin, not dirt;
(*c*) an increase in *Propionibacterium acnes* bacteria in the duct;
(*d*) an increase in free fatty acids;
(*e*) inflammation around the sebaceous gland; probably as a result of the release of bacterial enzymes.

Underlying causes

There are various underlying causes of these changes.
Hormones—Androgenic hormones increase the size of sebaceous glands and the amount of sebum in both male and female adolescents. Oestrogens have the opposite effect in prepubertal boys and eunuchs. In some women with acne there is lowering of the concentration of sex hormone binding globulin and a consequent increase in free testosterone concentrations. There is probably also a variable increase in androgen sensitivity. Oral contraceptives containing more than 50 μg ethinyloestradiol can make acne worse and the combined type may lower sex hormone binding globulin concentrations, leading to increased free testosterone. Infantile acne occurs in the first few months of life and may last some years. Apart from rare causes, such as adrenal hyperplasia or virilising tumours, transplacental stimulation of the adrenal gland is thought to result in the release of adrenal androgens—but this does not explain why the lesions persist. It is more common in boys.
Fluid retention—The premenstrual exacerbation of acne is thought to be due to fluid retention leading to increased hydration of and swelling of the duct. Sweating also makes acne worse, possibly by the same mechanism.

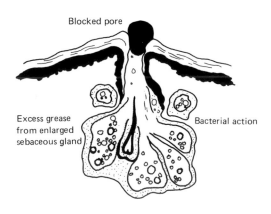

Blocked pore

Excess grease from enlarged sebaceous gland

Bacterial action

Diet—In some patients acne is made worse by chocolate, nuts, and coffee or fizzy drinks.

Seasons—Acne often improves with natural sunlight and is worse in winter. The effect of artificial ultraviolet light is unpredictable.

External factors—Oils, whether vegetable oils in the case of cooks in hot kitchens or mineral oils in engineering, can cause "oil folliculitis," leading to acne like lesions. Other acnegenic substances include coal tar, dicophane (DDT), cutting oils, and halogenated hydrocarbons (polychlorinated biphenols and related chemicals). Cosmetic acne is seen in adult women who have used cosmetics containing comedogenic oils over many years.

Iatrogenic—Corticosteroids, both topical and systemic, can cause increased keratinisation of the pilosebaceous duct. Androgens, gonadotrophins, and corticotrophin can induce acne in adolescence. Oral contraceptives of the combined type can induce acne, and antiepileptic drugs are reputed to cause acne.

Hormones—the cause of all the trouble	
Androgens	increase the size of sebaceous glands
	increase sebum secretion
Androgenic adrenocorticosteroids have the same effect	
Oestrogens	have the opposite effect

Types of acne

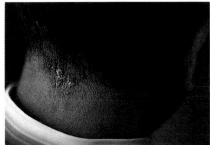

Acne keloidalis.

Acne vulgaris

Acne vulgaris, the common type of acne, occurs during puberty and affects the comedogenic areas of the face, back, and chest. There may be a familial tendency to acne. Acne vulgaris is slightly more common in boys, 30-40% of whom have acne between the ages of 18 and 19. In girls the peak incidence is between 16 and 18 years. Adult acne is a variant, affecting 1% of men and 5% of women aged 40. Acne keloidalis is a type of scarring acne seen on the neck in men.

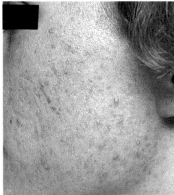

Patients with acne often complain of excessive greasiness of the skin, with "blackheads," "pimples," or "plukes" developing. These may be associated with inflammatory papules and pustules developing into larger cysts and nodules. Resolving lesions leave inflammatory macules and scarring. Scars may be atrophic, sometimes with "ice pick" lesions or keloid formation. Keloids consist of hypertrophic scar tissue and occur predominantly on the neck, upper back, and shoulders and over the sternum.

Infantile acne—Localised acne lesions occur on the face in the first few months of life. They clear spontaneously but may last for some years. There is said to be an associated increased tendency to severe adolescent acne.

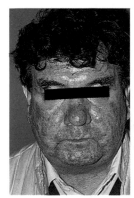
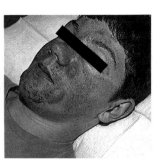
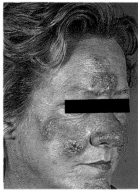

Acne conglobata—This is a severe form of acne, more common in boys and in tropical climates. It is extensive, affecting the trunk, face, and limbs. In "acne fulminans" there is associated systemic illness with malaise, fever, and joint pains. It appears to be associated with a hypersensitivity to *P acnes*. Another variant is pyoderma faciale, which produces erythematous and necrotic lesions and occurs mainly in adult women.

Acne conglobata.   Acne fulminans.   Pyoderma faciale.

Acne and Rosacea

Acne vulgaris

  affects comedogenic areas
  occurs mainly in puberty,
    in boys more than girls
  familial tendency

Infantile acne

  face only
  clears spontaneously

Severe acne

  acne conglobata
  pyoderma faciale
  Gram negative folliculitis

Occupational acne

  oils
  coal and tar
  chlorinated phenols
  DDT and weedkillers

Steroids

  systemic or topical

Hormones

  combined type of oral contraceptives
  androgenic hormones

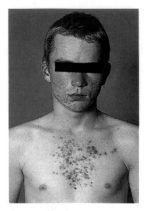

Acne vulgaris.

Gram negative folliculitis.

Gram negative folliculitis occurs with a proliferation of organisms such as klebsiella, proteus, pseudomonas, and *Escherichia coli*.

Occupational—Acne like lesions occur as a result of long term contact with oils or tar as mentioned above. This usually occurs as a result of lubricating, cutting, or crude oil soaking through clothing. In chloracne there are prominent comedones on the face and neck. It is caused by exposure to polychlortriphenyl and related compounds and also to weedkiller and dicophane.

Treatment of acne

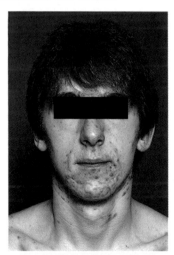

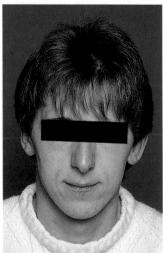

Before and after treatment with tetracycline.

In most adolescents acne clears spontaneously with minimal scarring. Reassurance and explanation along the following lines helps greatly.

(1) The lesions can be expected to clear in time.

(2) It is not infectious.

(3) The less are sufferers self conscious and worry about their appearance the less other people will take any notice of their acne.

It helps to give a simple regimen to follow, enabling patients to take some positive steps to clear their skin and also an alternative to picking their spots.

I advise patients with acne to hold a hot wet flannel on the face (a much simpler alternative to the commercial "facial saunas"), followed by gentle rubbing in of a plain soap. Savlon solution, diluted 10 times with water, is an excellent alternative for controlling greasy skin.

There are many proprietary preparations, most of which act as keratolytics, dissolving the keratin plug of the comedone. They can also cause considerable dryness and scaling of the skin.

Benzoyl peroxide in concentrations of 1% to 10% comes as lotions, creams, gels, and washes. Resorcinol, sulphur, and salicylic acid preparations are also available.

Vitamin A acid as a cream or gel is helpful in some patients.

Ultraviolet light therapy is less effective than natural sunlight but is helpful for extensive acne.

Oral treatment—The mainstay of treatment is oxytetracycline, which should be given for a week at 1 g daily then 500 mg (250 mg twice daily) on an empty stomach. Minocycline or doxycycline are alternatives that can be taken with food. Perseverance with treatment is important, and it may take some months to produce an appreciable improvement. Erythromycin is an alternative to tetracycline, and co-trimoxazole can be used for Gram negative folliculitis. Tetracycline might theoretically interfere with the action of progesterone types of birth control pill and should not be given in pregnancy.

Topical antibiotics—Erythromycin, the tetracyclines, and clindamycin have been used topically. There is the risk of producing colonies of resistant organisms.

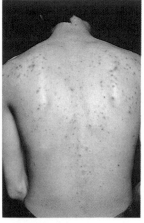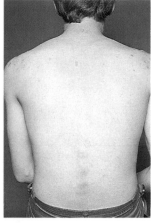

Before and after treatment with ultraviolet light.

Antiandrogens—Cyproterone acetate combined with ethinyloestradiol is effective in some women; it is also a contraceptive.

Synthetic retinoids—For severe cases resistant to other treatments these drugs, which can be prescribed only in hospital, are very effective and clear most cases in a few months. 13-*cis*-Retinoic acid (isotretinoin) is usually used for acne. They are teratogenic, so there must be no question of pregnancy, and can cause liver changes with raised serum lipid values. Regular blood tests are therefore essential. A three month course of treatment usually gives a long remission.

Ultraviolet light is a helpful additional treatment in the winter months.

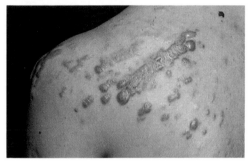

Keloid scars.

Residual lesions, keloid scars, cysts, and persistent nodules can be treated by injection with triamcinolone or freezing with liquid nitrogen. For severe scarring dermabrasion can produce good cosmetic results. This is usually carried out in a plastic surgery unit.

Remember the following points

(1) Avoid topical steroids
(2) Persevere with one antibiotic not short courses of different types
(3) Do not prescribe a tetracycline for children and pregnant women
(4) Oxytetracycline must be taken on an empty stomach half an hour before meals

---

Treatment of acne

First line	Second line
(1) Encourage positive attitudes	(1) Topical vitamin A acid
(2) Avoid environmental and occupational factors	(2) Topical antibiotics
(3) Topical treatment 　　Benzoyl peroxide 　　Salicylic acid	(3) Ultraviolet light
	(4) Antiandrogens
(4) A tetracycline by mouth for several months	*Third line*
	Oral retinoids for 3-4 months (hospitals only)

Rosacea

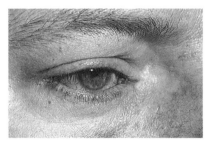

Blepharitis.

Rosacea is a persistent eruption occurring on the forehead and cheeks. It is more common in women than men.

There is erythema with prominent blood vessels. Pustules, papules, and oedema occur. Rhinophyma, with thickened erythematous skin of the nose and enlarged follicles, is a variant. Conjunctivitis and blepharitis may be associated. It is usually made worse by sunlight.

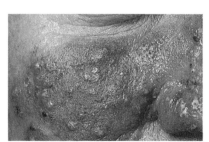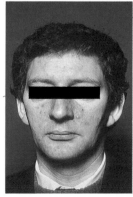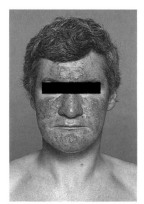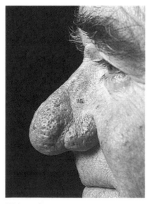

Rosacea.　　　　Rosacea.　　　　Rosacea.　　　　Rhinophyma.

Acne and Rosacea

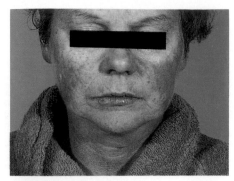

Lupus erythematosus.

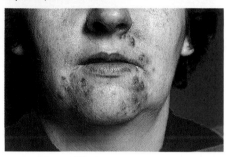

Perioral dermatitis.

Rosacea should be distinguished from:

Acne, in which there are blackheads, a wider distribution, and improvement with sunlight. Acne, however, may coexist with rosacea—hence the older term "acne rosacea";

Seborrhoeic eczema, in which there are no pustules and eczematous changes are present;

Lupus erythematosus, which shows light sensitivity, erythema, and scarring but no pustules;

Perioral dermatitis, which occurs in women with pustules and erythema around the mouth and on the chin. There is usually a premenstrual exacerbation. Treatment is with oral tetracyclines.

Treatment

The treatment of rosacea is with long term courses of oxytetracycline, which may need to be repeated. Topical treatment along the lines of that for acne is also helpful. Topical steroids should not be used as they have minimal effect and cause a severe rebound erythema, which is difficult to clear. Avoiding hot and spicy foods may help.

Recent reports indicate that synthetic retinoids are also effective.

BACTERIAL INFECTION

The process of infection involves the interaction of two organisms—host and invader. The clinical changes are a manifestation of the resulting "battle of the cells" as so clearly perceived by Metchnikoff 100 years ago. The lesions produced may have a well recognised appearance, such as impetigo or tinea cruris, but are often less specific.

Several features enable us to recognise that infection is a possible cause of the patient's condition.

Acute bacterial infections produce the classical characteristics of acute inflammation described by Celsus (see box).

> ***Rubor***—erythema
> ***Tumor***—swelling and oedema
> ***Calor***—heat or warmth
> ***Dolor***—pain and discomfort

Presentation

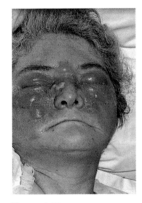
Presentation.

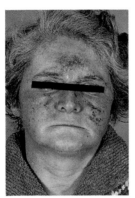
Two weeks later.

This woman had acute *erysipelas* due to a haemolytic streptococcus, and all four features were present. She was, however, referred to the clinic with a diagnosis of acute allergy, which, from the appearance alone, was understandable. However, malaise and fever were also present and the lesions were warm. The condition responded well to antibiotic treatment. The point of entry in such cases may be a "spot" on the face or a small erosion near the nose, mouth, or ears. Erysipelas of the leg or foot may follow a small fissure between the toes.

Erysipelas is the local manifestation of a streptococcal infection, but this organism in the throat can result in the widespread rash of scarlet fever, which is rarely seen these days, or erythema multiforme, which is more common. An acute generalised vasculitis can also be associated with a streptococcal infection.

More chronic forms of bacterial infection include *impetigo, folliculitis, carbuncles,* and *ecthyma*. These conditions are due to streptococci and particularly to staphylococci, which are adept at colonising the skin, commonly in those with atopic eczema. Bacterial infection occurs in eczematous lesions and may itself cause an exacerbation of eczema.

Impetigo is a superficial infection of the skin, with transient blisters in the non-bullous form that then form crusts. Both staphylococci and streptococci are responsible. The bullous form is due to staphylococci.

Folliculitis, with infection and inflammatory changes in the upper follicle, is common. Deeper forms occur in the scalp (follicular impetigo) or the beard area (sycosis barbae). Abscess formation in the hair follicles results in furuncles or boils—confluent lesions forming a carbuncle.

Ecthyma, which is most common on the leg, is due to bacterial infection causing a nectrotic lesion with a superficial crust and surrounding inflammation. Both streptococci and staphylococci are responsible.

(1) In any patient with a localised area of acute erythema, swelling, and raised temperature consider infection.

(2) Remember that a *generalised* erythematous rash may be the manifestation of a *localised* infection. Scarlet fever arises from streptococcal throat infection, and herpes simplex of the lip may be associated with erythema multiforme.

(3) The common pathogens are also commensals—recent studies showed that 60% of individuals are nasal carriers of *Staphylococcus aureus* intermittently and 10% carry *Streptococcus pyogenes* in the throat.

Bacterial infection
Common patterns of cutaneous bacterial infection

	Infected eczema	*Impetigo (non-bullous)*	*Impetigo (bullous)*
Appearance	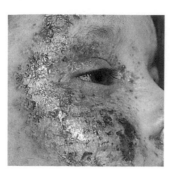	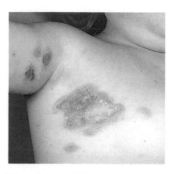	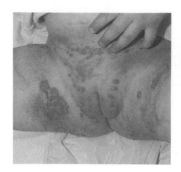
	Exudate Crusts Inflammation	Transient vesicles Exuding lesions with yellow crusts Erythema Affects mainly face and limbs, commonly in children	Erythema and bullae which rupture to leave superficial crusts May be central clearing Affects face, buttocks, and limbs in children and adults
Cause	Persistent scratching Topical steroids	Local reaction between invading organisms and neutrophils, resulting in superficial epidermal split in bullous lesion	
Organism	*Staphylococcus aureus* *Streptococcus pyogenes*	*Staphylococcus aureus* *Streptococcus pyogenes* in some outbreaks	*Staphylococcus aureus*
Treatment	(1) Weaker topical steroids (for the eczema) with topical antibiotics (2) Systemic antibiotics if necessary (3) Soaks with potassium permanganate (4) 1% eosin or gentian violet to paint erosions	Topical antibiotics Systemic antibiotics directed against both streptococcal and staphylococcal infection	Topical and systemic antibiotics
Notes	● Avoid prolonged use of topical antibiotics ● Return to using weaker steroid when infection has healed ● Even without clinical evidence of infection most lesions of atopic eczema are colonised by *Staphylococcus aureus*	● Staphylococcal infection can cause widespread superficial shedding of the epidermis—"scalded skin syndrome" (Lyell's disease) ● It is wise to send a specimen for bacteriology: nephritogenic strains of streptococcus in impetigo remain an important cause for glomerulonephritis, although this is a rare condition.	

Boils (and furuncles) and carbuncles	***Folliculitis***	***Ecthyma***	***Erysipelas***
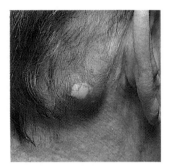	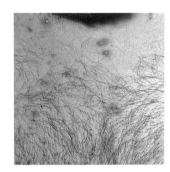	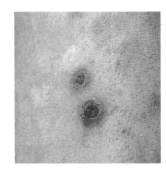	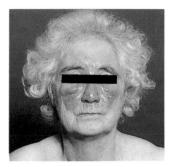
Inflammatory nodule affecting the hair follicles develops into a pustule Tender induration with considerable inflammation, followed by necrosis Heals with scarring More common in adolescents in winter Several boils may coalesce to form a carbuncle	Various forms: (1) *Scalp* *Children*—"Follicular impetigo" *Adults*— (*a*) Folliculitis cheloidalis Back of neck (*b*) Acne necrotica Forehead/hairline (2) *Face*—"Sycosis barbae" in men with seborrhoea (greasy skin) (3) *Legs*—Chronic folliculitis	Small bullae may be present initially An adherent crust is followed by a purulent ulcerated lesion with surrounding erythema and induration, which slowly heals Usually on legs	Well defined areas of erythema—very tender, not oedematous Vesicles may form Common sites—abdominal wall in infants; in adults the lower leg and face An area of broken skin, forming a portal of entry, may be found
Possible anaemia and fatigue Mechanical damage from clothing	(1) Underlying disease—eg diabetes (2) Infection may be precipitated by mechanical injury, tar pastes, and occlusive dressings	Minor injuries More common in debilitated individuals	Lymphoedema and severe inflammation due to bacterial toxins
Staphylococcus aureus, usually of same strain as in nose and perineum	*Staphylococcus aureus* *Propionibacterium acnes* *Pityrosporum* spp *Pseudomonas* spp and other Gram negative organisms	Both streptococcus and staphylococcus	*Streptococcus pyogenes* (group A, but may be B, C, or G) *Staphylococcus aureus* *Klebsiella pneumoniae* *Haemophilus influenzae*
(1) Antibiotic (penicillinase resistant) systemically (2) Cleaning of skin with weak chlorhexedine solution or a similar preparation	Topical and long term systemic antibiotics—eg oxytetracycline Topical antifungal for pityrosporum infection	Improve nutrition Use antibiotic effective against both staphylococcus and streptococcus	Penicillin or erythromycin
● Nasal and perineal swabs should be taken to identify carriers ● Remember unusual causes—a bricklayer presented with a boil on the arm with necrosis due to anthrax (malignant pustule) acquired from the packing straw used for the bricks	● Gram negative folliculitis occurs on the face—a complication of long term treatment for acne ● A persistent, painful type of necrotic folliculitis occurs in those who wear hats, caps, or helmets for long periods	● Check for debilitating diseases, reticuloses, diabetes	● Cellulitis affects the deeper tissues and has more diverse causes, being essentially inflammation of the connective tissue ● Streptococcus, staphylococcus, haemophilus, and other organisms may be found ● Beware of erysipelas of the face—the venous drainage is deep to the cavernous sinus. A young resident physician decided to "tough out" her erysipelas on the cheek and refused treatment. Severe fever, facial oedema, and malaise associated with cavernous sinus phlebitis followed

Bacterial infection
Mycobacterial disease

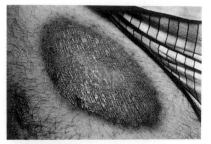

Lupus vulgaris.

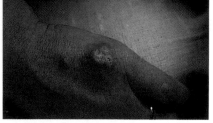

Swimming pool granuloma.

The clinical presentation of mycobacterial disease depends on the immune response of the host—hence the difference between disseminated miliary tuberculosis and lupus vulgaris or, for example, tuberculoid and lepromatous leprosy.

These infections are rarely seen in the West so only the most common types—lupus vulgaris and "atypical mycobacterial infection" are described.

Lupus vulgaris is a very slowly growing indolent condition of the skin. The lesion shown had been present for 20 years and may have been acquired from the cattle with which the man worked. The characteristic giant cell granuloma can be clearly seen.

Atypical mycobacterial infections—Although infection with *Mycobacterium tuberculosis* is now rare in Britain, other types of mycobacterial skin infection occur. The most common is "fishtank" or "swimming pool" granuloma, acquired from tropical fish tackle or swimming pools, respectively, and caused by *Mycobacterium marinum*. Nodular lesions develop slowly with ulceration but there is no regional lymph node enlargement. *Mycobacterium kansasii* infection is rare and *Mycobacterium ulcerans* confined to the tropics.

Erythema of the face

Acute

	Usually unilateral	Usually bilateral	Photosensitive
(1) Allergic reactions			
Cosmetics (*left*)		+	+ or −
Plants	+	or +	+ or −
Drugs		+	+ or −
(2) Urticaria		+	−
Reactions to light			
(3) Photodermatitis (*right*)		+	+
Solar urticaria		+	+
(4) Infection			
Erysipelas (*left*)		+	−
Fifth disease ("slapped cheek")		+	−
(5) Rosacea (*right*)		+	+ or −

Chronic-recurrent

	Usually unilateral	Usually bilateral	Photosensitive
(6) Lupus erythematosus			
Systemic (*left*)		+	+
Discoid (*right*)	+	or +	+
(7) Seborrhoeic dermatitis (*left*)		+	−
(8) Acne		+	+
(9) Perioral dermatitis (*right*)		+	−

VIRAL INFECTIONS

Herpes

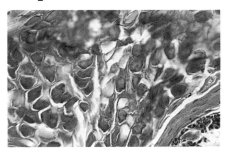
Herpes virus inclusion bodies.

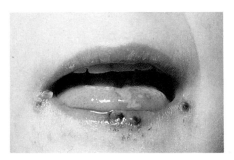
Herpes of lips.

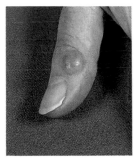
Inoculation herpes.

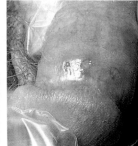
Genital herpes.

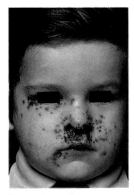
Eczema herpeticum.

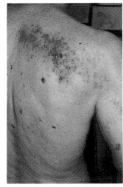

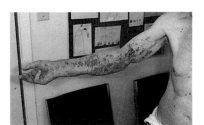
Herpes zoster.

Like the pyogenic bacteria, viruses produce local lesions and may cause a widespread reaction to the infection. The clinical manifestations of common viral infections of the skin are well known and easily recognised.

Local infective lesions are caused by DNA viruses which can be isolated from the lesions themselves and include the herpes and pox groups.

Herpes simplex

The herpes simplex virus consists of two antigenic types. Type I is associated with lesions on the face and fingers and sometimes genital lesions. Type II is associated almost entirely with genital infections.

Primary herpes simplex (type I) infection, usually occurs in or around the mouth, with variable involvement of the face. Although there is usually a small area of inflammation with irritation forming a vesicle, there may be considerable inflammation and necrosis with malaise, probably depending on the degree of protection from maternal antibodies. Subsequent recurrent chronic infection of the lips may be due to virus remaining in the sensory nerve ganglia.

Type II infection affects the genitalia, vagina, and cervix and may predispose to cervical dysplasia.

● The initial vesicular stage may not be seen in genital lesions, which present as painful ulcers or erosions.

● There is usually a history of preceding itching and tenderness.

● Scrapings from the base of the ulcer can be stained for viral inclusion bodies (Tzanck smears). Viral antigen can be shown by immunofluorescence.

● Genital herpes in a pregnant woman carries a great risk of ophthalmic infection of the infant. Caesarean section may be indicated.

● "Eczema herpeticum" or "Kaposi's varicelliform eruption" are terms applied to lifethreatening systemic infection with herpes virus in patients with atopic eczema and some other skin conditions. Treatment is with parenteral acyclovir. It can also be caused by vaccinia and coxsackie viruses.

Herpes zoster

Herpes zoster, due to herpesvirus varicella, which also causes chickenpox (due to a herpes virus, not a pox virus), develops without a definable incubation period. There is, however, often pain, fever, and malaise before erythematous papules develop in the area of the affected dermatome—most commonly in the thoracic area. Vesicles develop over several days, leaving dried crusts as they resolve. Secondary infection is common. The subsequent neuralgia, particularly in elderly individuals, is well known.

● Trigeminal zoster may occur and affect the ophthalmic nerve (causing severe conjunctivitis); the maxillary nerve (causing vesicles on the uvula or tonsils); or the mandibular nerve (causing vesicles on the floor of the mouth and on the tongue).

● Visceral lesions can occur with pleuritic and abdominal pain.

● Disseminated zoster is a severe illness, often with haemorrhagic lesions.

Viral infections

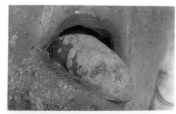
Mandibular zoster.

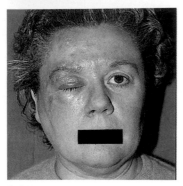
Ophthalmic zoster.

Pox viruses

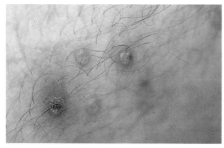
Molluscum contagiosum.

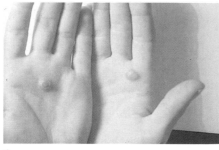
Cowpox.

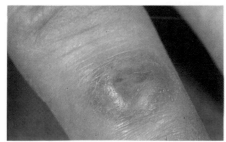
Milkers' node.

Remember that infection from both skin lesions and nasopharyngeal secretions can cause chickenpox.

Treatment

The usual troublesome, localised lesions of herpes simplex have been treated with topical zinc sulphate, iodoxuridine, ice cubes, and photoactivation of eosin. Topical acyclovir—a drug that inhibits herpes virus DNA polymerase—is effective and should be used as soon as the patient is aware of symptoms.

Severe, recurrent, herpes simplex or herpes zoster can be treated with acyclovir by mouth or injection, given as early in the course of the illness as possible.

Secondary infection may require antiseptic soaks, such as 1/1000 potassium permanganate, or topical or systemic antibiotics.

Steroids (prednisolone 40-60 mg/day) given during the acute stage of herpes zoster diminish pain and postherpetic neuralgia.

Rest and analgesics are recommended treatment for extensive herpes simplex or herpes zoster infections.

> Steroids should not be given to immunodeficient patients, in whom they may cause disseminated infection

The pox viruses are also large DNA viruses, particularly infecting the epidermis.

Variola (smallpox), once the cause of high mortality, has been officially eliminated by vaccination with modified vaccinia virus—the culmination of Jenner's pioneer work.

Molluscum contagiosum

The commonest "pox" seen these days is molluscum contagiosum—a worry to mothers of affected infants, who are not themselves unduly concerned. Despite its name it is not very contagious, except in overcrowded conditions in tropical countries. In temperate climates it often affects only one or two children in a household.

Clinical features—The white, umbilicated papules of molluscum contagiosum are characteristic. Large solitary lesions may cause confusion and so can secondarily infected, excoriated lesions. Remember that these can itch, particularly in patients with atopy. There may be widespread lesions, which are said to be more common in sarcoidosis and atopy. I have seen several episodes in adults after open heart surgery.

Diagnosis is not difficult. Sometimes there is confusion with viral warts and benign tumours of the skin.

Treatment—Most treatments are painful and should not be inflicted on a child with a benign self limiting condition. An antibiotic-hydrocortisone ointment can be used for excoriated lesions. Treatment with liquid nitrogen is probably the simplest treatment. Other methods include superficial curettage and rotating a sharpened orange stick moistened with phenol in the centre of each lesion.

Other pox infections

The other pox infections are of incidental interest.

Cowpox only sporadically infects cows from its natural reservoir, probably small mammals, and may affect man.

Milkers' nodules are due to a virus that causes superficial ulcers in cows' udders and calves' mouths. In humans papules on the hands develop into grey nodules with a necrotic centre, surrounding inflammation, and lymphangeitis. A more generalised papular eruption can occur.

Orf is easily diagnosed by country doctors, sheep farmers, and veterinarians but may be overinvestigated by those less familiar with rural dermatology. It is seen mainly in early spring as a result of contact with lambs. A single papule or group of lesions develops on the fingers or hands

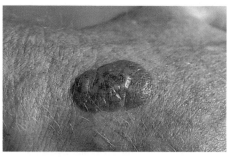

Orf.

with purple papules developing into a bulla. This ruptures to leave a varied annular lesion 1-3 cm in diameter with a necrotic centre. There is surrounding inflammation. The incubation period is a few days and the lesions last 2-3 weeks with spontaneous healing. Associated erythema multiforme and widespread rashes are occasionally seen.

Monkey pox, reindeer pox, and *musk ox pox* are of interest to those treating zookeepers and travellers.

Wart viruses

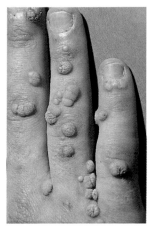

Common warts.

The true worth of the papilloma virus, which causes warts, as an object of serious study has only recently been recognised. The wart is, after all, one of the few tumours in which a virus can be seen to proliferate in the cell nucleus. The different types of wart caused by the many different types of papilloma viruses cannot be discussed here but certain aspects should be remembered.

(1) Genital warts (due to human papilloma virus) very rarely undergo malignant change but the associated infection of the cervix frequently leads to dysplasia or malignant changes. Cervical smears must be taken.

(2) Very extensive proliferation of warts occurs in patients receiving immunosuppressive therapy, such as renal transplant recipients.

(3) Epidermodysplasia verruciformis, an unusual widespread eruption of erythematous warty plaques, can develop into carcinoma.

Treatment

Most warts occur in children and resolve spontaneously without treatment or with very simple measures. These include paints or lotions containing salicylic and lactic acid and formalin in various proportions, which should be applied daily. Salicylic acid (40%) plasters are useful for plantar warts; they are cut to shape and held in place with sticking plaster for two or three days. Glutaraldehyde solution is also used.

For warts that get in the way, are painful, or are disfiguring more drastic measures can be used.

(1) *Cold*—Carbon dioxide snow is readily produced from a cylinder and can be mixed with acetone to form a slush. This is applied with a cotton wool swab. Liquid nitrogen is colder and more effective but has to be stored in special containers and replaced frequently. It can be applied with cotton wool or discharged from a special spray apparatus. Freezing is continued until there is a rim of frozen tissue around the wart but not for more than 30 seconds. Subsequent blistering may occur. Scarring is unusual.

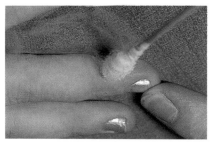

Treatment.

(2) *Heat*—Cautery causes more scarring and requires local anaesthesia.

(3) *Curettage and cautery* together are effective but leave scars and the warts may recur.

(4) *Podophyllin*, 15% in tincture of benzoin compound, is effective for genital warts when applied each week. It is, however, toxic when ingested or absorbed and must never be used in pregnancy.

Other treatments include radiotherapy, fluorouracil, and bleomycin injections. Hypnosis has been effectively used, and fear of painful treatment has caused warts to fall off.

Virus diseases with rashes

Measles
Rubella
Infectious mononucleosis
Erythema infectiosum
Roseola infantum
Gianotti-Crosti syndrome
Hand, foot, and mouth disease

Measles and rubella, which were once familiar to every doctor, are now much less common as a result of widespread inoculation. However, measles is probably the best known example of an exanthem (a fever characterised by a skin eruption. In an enanthem the mucous surfaces are affected). Other common clinical patterns can then be compared with it. All exanthems, except fifth disease (erythema infectiosum), are due to RNA viruses.

Viral infections

Measles

Age—Measles affects children, usually those aged over 5.
Incubation lasts seven to 14 days.
Prodromal symptoms include fever, malaise, upper respiratory symptoms; conjunctivitis; and photophobia.
Initial rash—Early on Koplik's spots (white spots with surrounding erythema) appear on the oral mucosa. After two days a macular rash appears on the face, trunk, and limbs. Look behind the ears for early lesions.
Development and resolution—The rash becomes papular, with coalescence. There may be haemorrhagic lesions and bullae which fade to leave brown patches.
Complications are encephalitis, otitis media, and bronchopneumonia.
Diagnosis—Specific antibodies may be detected; they are at their maximum at two to four weeks.

Rubella

Age—Rubella affects children and young adults.
Incubation lasts 14 to 21 days.
Prodromal symptoms—There are none in young children. Otherwise fever, malaise, and upper respiratory symptoms occur.
Initial rash—Initially some patients develop erythema of the soft palate and lymphadenopathy. Later pink macules appear on the face, spreading to trunk and limbs over one to two days.
Development and resolution—The rash then clears over the next two days, and sometimes no rash develops at all.
Complications—The main complication is congenital defects in babies of women infected during pregnancy. The risk is greatest in the first month.
Diagnosis—The diagnosis is made from the clinical signs above. Serum should be taken for measuring antibodies and the test repeated at seven to 10 days.
Prophylaxis—Active immunisation is now routinely available for all schoolgirls.

Erythema infectiosum (fifth disease)

Age group—Erythema infectiosum affects children aged 2-10 years, mainly girls.
Incubation lasts five to 20 days.
Prodromal symptoms—There are usually none, but there may be a slight fever with initial rash.
Initial rash—The initial rash is a hot, erythematous eruption on the cheeks—hence the "slapped cheek syndrome." Over two to four days a maculopapular eruption develops on the arms, legs, and trunk.
Development and resolution—The rash extends to affect hands, feet, and mucous membranes, then fades over one to two weeks.
Diagnosis is made by finding a specific IgM antibody to parvovirus B19.
Complications—There are no reported dermatological complications but haematological disorders, arthropathy, and fetal abnormalities may be associated.

Roseola infantum

Age group—Roseola infantum affects infants aged under 2.
Incubation lasts 10-15 days.
Prodromal symptoms—There is fever for a few days.
Initial rash—A rose pink maculopapular eruption appears on the neck and trunk.

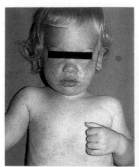
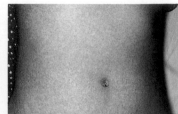
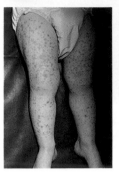
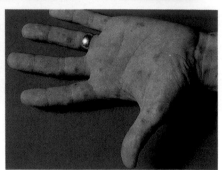

Measles (left); rubella (below); Gianotti-Crosti syndrome (below left); hand, foot, and mouth disease (below right).

Development and resolution—The rash may affect the face and limbs before clearing over one to two days.
Diagnosis—The condition is diagnosed from its clinical features.
Complications include febrile convulsions.

Gianotti-Crosti syndrome

Age group—The Gianotti-Crosti syndrome affects children, usually those aged under 14.
Incubation period is unknown.
Prodromal symptoms—Lymphadenopathy and malaise accompany the eruption.
Initial rash—Red papules rapidly develop on the face, neck, limbs, buttocks, palms, and soles.
Development and resolution—Over two to three weeks the lesions become purpuric then slowly fade.
Diagnosis—The syndrome may be due to a number of virus infections. Check for hepatitis B antigen.
Complications—Lymphadenopathy and hepatomegaly always occur and may persist for many months.

Hand, foot, and mouth disease

Age—Hand, foot, and mouth disease (Coxsackie virus A) affects both children and adults.
Incubation period is unknown.
Prodromal symptoms—Fever, headache, and malaise may accompany the rash.
Initial rash—Initially there may be intense erythema surrounding yellow-grey vesicles; ulceration then occurs. This pattern is more common in adults. Alternatively, there may be grey vesicles, 1-5 mm diameter, with surrounding erythema on the palms and soles. These occur mainly in children, in whom a more generalised eruption may develop.
Development and resolution—Over three to five days the rash fades.
Diagnosis—Coxsackie A (usually A16) virus is isolated from lesions and stools. A specific antibody may be found in the serum.
Complications are rare but include widespread vesicular rashes and erythema multiforme.

Other infections

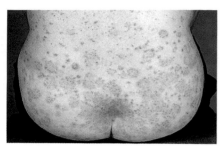

Secondary syphilis.

Infectious mononucleosis—As well as the erythematous lesions on the palate a maculopapular rash affecting the face and limbs can occur.

Cat scratch disease—A crusted nodule at the site of the scratch is associated with development of regional lymphadenopathy one to two months later. A maculopapular eruption on the face and limbs or erythema multiforme may occur.

Psittacosis and ornithosis may be associated with a rash.

Rickettsial infections, including typhus, Rocky Mountain spotted fever, and Rickettsial pox are all associated with rashes.

Syphilis—Although not a viral infection, the transient roseolar rash of secondary syphilis is followed by a papulosquamous eruption, which affects the trunk, limbs, and mucous membranes. The palms and soles may be affected. The diagnosis should always be considered in any rash that does not fit a recognised pattern.

The photographs of herpes of the lips, measles, and rubella are reproduced by kind permission of Dr A P Ball.

FUNGAL AND YEAST INFECTIONS

Fungal infections

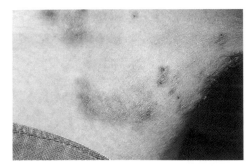

T rubrum infection of the neck.

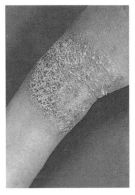

Animal ringworm.

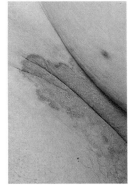

Tinea cruris.

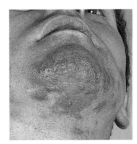

T mentagrophytes.

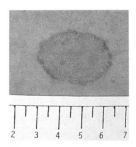

M canis.

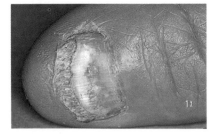

Fungal infection of nail.

Fungal infections are commonly known as "ringworm"—a misnomer since most infections cause a scaling macule, not a ring, and the worm exists only in the imagination. It is true, however, that a superficial fungal infection can have a raised edge, and annular forms occur.

Fungi consist of thread-like hyphae—which form tangled masses, or mycelia, in the common moulds. In superficial fungal infection of the skin, hair, and nails it is these hyphae that invade keratin and are seen on microscopic examination of keratin from infected tissues. Vegetative spores (conidia) develop in culture, and their distinctive shape helps to differentiate one species from another. "Dermatophyte" fungi include the common species that invade hair, skin, and nails.

Systemic, or deep, fungal infection is due to those species that invade other tissues. When the immune response is impaired superficial infections may invade the deeper tissues.

Yeasts are budding unicellular organisms that do not normally produce hyphae. The commonest infective species in man is *Candida albicans*.

Why should one suspect a lesion to be due to a fungus?

Clinical presentation

Fungal infections usually itch. Those due to zoophilic (animal) fungi produce a more intense inflammatory response with deeper indurated lesions than those due to anthropophilic (human) species. In those lesions with a raised scaling margin that extends outwards the fungal hyphae are invading the keratin layer in this area. The central area is relatively resistant to colonisation. Such lesions occur mainly on the trunk.

Children below the age of puberty rarely develop anthropophilic (human) fungal infection. In the countryside cattle ringworm (zoophilic) infects children in the autumn when the cows are brought into winter quarters. Pet mice can be a source of infection.

Adults—From adolescence onwards infection of the feet, not only in athletes, occurs. Tinea cruris in the groin is seen mainly in men.

Infection from cattle occurs in adults who have not had previous exposure, sometimes in unusual ways. A man who lived in an industrial area housing estate developed a curious indurated lesion on his chin from which *Trichophyton mentagrophytes* was isolated—transmitted by bites from midges who had been biting cows on a farm some miles away.

Infection from dogs and cats with a zoophilic fungus (*Microsporum canis*) to which humans have little immunity can occur at any age. A colleague's daughter returned from a skiing holiday with intensely itchy "eczema," which refused to clear. A stray kitten, mewing outside in the dark, had been taken indoors, warmed in their sleeping bags, and infected the whole party with *M canis*.

Nail infections occur mainly in adults, usually in their toenails, especially when traumatised—for example, the big toes of footballers. The nails become thickened and yellow and crumble, usually asymmetrically. The changes occur *distally* and move back to the nailfold. In psoriasis of the nail the changes occur *proximally* and tend to be symmetrical and are associated with pitting and other evidence of psoriasis elsewhere. Chronic

Fungal and yeast infections

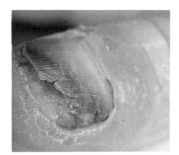

Chronic paronychia.

paronychia occurs in the fingers of individuals whose work demands repeated wetting of the hands: housewives, barmen, dentists, nurses, and mushroom growers, for example. There is erythema and swelling of the nail fold, often on one side with brownish discoloration of the nail. Pus may be exuded. The cause is *Candida albicans* (a yeast) together with secondary bacterial infection. The hands should be kept as dry as possible, nystatin cream applied regularly, and, if necessary, a course of erythromycin prescribed.

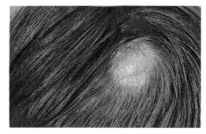

Tinea pedis.

Feet—It is not only athletes and the unhygienic who suffer from athletes' foot but increased sweating does predispose to infection. The hands may be affected, often through scratching the feet; hence the "right hand, left foot" syndrome in the right handed individual. The itching, macerated skin beneath the toes is familiar, but when a dry, scaling rash extends across the sole and dorsal surface of one foot the diagnosis may be missed. The condition needs to be differentiated from psoriasis and eczema.

Hands—Fungal infections often produce a dry, hot, rash on one palm. There may be well defined lesions with a scaling edge.

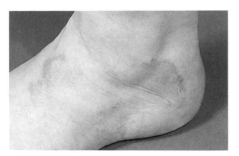

Tinea corporis. Erythrasma.

Trunk—Tinea corporis presents with erythema and itching and a well defined scaling edge. The infection may spread to the adjacent skin on the thighs and abdomen. Intense erythema and satellite lesions suggests a candida infection. In the axillae erythrasma due to *Corynebacterium minutissimum* is more likely. It does not respond to antifungal treatment but clears with tetracycline by mouth.

"Tinea incognita" is the term used for unrecognised fungal infection in patients treated with steroids (topical or systemic). The normal response to infection (leading to erythema, scaling, a raised margin, and itching) is diminished, particularly with local steroid creams or ointments. The infecting organism flourishes, however, because of the host's impaired immune response—shown by the enlarging, persistent skin lesions. The groins, hands, and face are sites where this is most likely to occur.

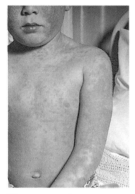

M audouini.

Scalp and face—The classic scalp ringworm of children due to *Microsporum audouini* is rare. Favus, a scarring type of alopecia, caused by *Trichophyton schoenleini*, and "black dot" ringworm, also from a trichophyton, are now seen only in children who have acquired the infection abroad. In all cases there is itching, hair loss, and some degree of inflammation. *M canis* from dogs and cats can affect the scalp.

Kerion—an inflamed, boggy, pustular lesion, is due to cattle ringworm and is fairly common in rural areas. It is often seen in children in the autumn when the cows are brought inside for the winter.

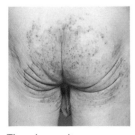
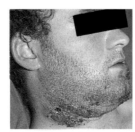

Tinea incognita. Actinomycosis.

Deep fungal infection

Fungal infection of the deeper tissues is rare in the United Kingdom but is of course a feature of the acquired immune deficiency syndrome. The species that colonise the deep tissue, as in histoplasmosis, actinomycosis, and cryptococcosis, can also cause skin lesions. In any patient with chronic indurated inflammatory lesions the possibility of deep fungal infection should be considered.

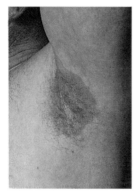

Fungal and yeast infections

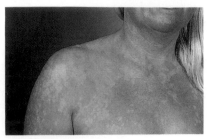

Tinea versicolor.

Tinea versicolor affects the trunk, usually of fair skinned individuals exposed to the sun. It affects mainly the upper back, chest, and arms. Well defined macular lesions with fine scales develop which tend to be white in suntanned areas and brown on pale skin (hence "versicolor"—variable colour). It may be confused with seborrhoeic dermatitis, pityriasis rosea, and vitiligo.

In skin scrapings the causative organism, *Pityrosporum* spp—normally found in hair follicles—can be readily seen.

Yeast infections

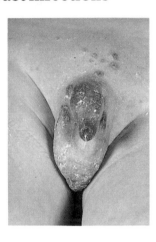

Candida albicans.

Candida infection may occur in the flexures of infants and elderly or immobilised patients, especially below the breasts and folds of abdominal skin. It needs to be differentiated from (a) psoriasis, which does not itch; (b) seborrhoeic dermatitis, the usual cause of a flexural rash in infants; and (c) contact dermatitis and discoid eczema, which do not have the scaling margin. It is symmetrical.

Yeasts, including *Candida albicans*, may be found in the mouth and vagina of healthy individuals. Clinical lesions may be produced by local trauma predisposing factors including: general debilitation, impaired immunity, diabetes mellitus, endocrine disorders, particularly Cushing's syndrome, and corticosteroid treatment. Florid mucocutaneous lesions can occur in which mycelial forms of *Candida albicans* are found.

Principles of diagnosis and treatment

(1) Consider a fungal infection in any patient where isolated, itching, dry, and scaling lesions occur without any apparent reason—for example, if there is no previous history of eczema. Lesions due to fungal infection are often asymmetrical.

(2) Skin scrapings should be sent to the laboratory from any suspicious lesion and are easy to take. The skin scales should be removed by scraping the edge of the lesion with a scalpel at right angles to the skin on to a piece of folded black paper. A strip of Sellotape applied to the lesion then stuck on a slide gives the laboratory more material for culture. Some laboratories supply mycology kits containing black paper, a slide with Sellotape, and suitable plastic containers. Clippings can be taken from the nails.

(3) Lesions to which steroids have been applied are often quite atypical because the normal inflammatory response is suppressed—tinea incognita. The patient often states that the treatment controls the itch but the contagion lingers on, becoming worse when the steroid is stopped. This may also occur in eczema being treated with steroids.

(4) Wood's light (ultraviolet light filtered through special glass) can be used to show microsporum infections, which produce a green-blue fluorescence.

Treatment

The old fashioned treatment with Whitfield's ointment (benzoic acid ointment, compound *BPC*) is quite effective, but has been superseded by the new imidazole preparations, such as clotrimazole and miconazole. The polyenes, nystatin and amphotericin, do not affect fungal infection but are effective against yeast infection. For damp macerated skin dusting powders or painting with Castellani's paint (magenta paint *BPC*) is helpful.

Systemic treatment is with griseofulvin, which should be taken for an adequate length of time: three to four months for the trunk and scalp, six to eight months for finger nails, and at least a year for toenails, where it is often ineffective. It is important to confirm the diagnosis from scrapings before starting treatment. The dose is 500 mg daily for adults and 10 mg/kg for children (taken with food).

Contraindications to griseofulvin are pregnancy, liver failure, and porphyria. It interacts with the coumarin anticoagulants, and its effect is diminished with barbiturates. Ketoconazole is an effective second choice but side effects may occur and are still being assessed.

INSECT BITES AND INFESTATIONS

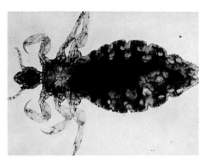

Body louse.

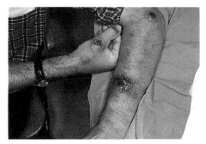

Leishmaniasis.

So, naturalists observe, a flea
Hath smaller fleas that on him prey;
And these have smaller fleas to bite 'em
And so proceed "Ad infinitum."

JONATHAN SWIFT

It is, of course, the internal parasites of biting insects that cause trouble for man, rather than "smaller fleas" on their surface.

An ornithologist went bird watching in Guyana, where he sustained widespread "midge bites" on the arms. He was referred on account of nodules that developed a few weeks later, then enlarged and ulcerated. Other lesions occurred further up the arms with regional lymphadenopathy. A biopsy specimen showed histiocytic inflammatory changes, and *Leishmania braziliensis* was isolated from smears; the midges (*phlebotomus* or sand fly) had acquired the protozoon while feeding on local rodents and transferred it into the ornithologist's skin.

Serious disease from insect vectors is rare in residents of most Western countries but, as in the patient described above, must be considered in those returning from tropical and subtropical countries.

Most cases of bites from fleas, midges, and mosquitoes are readily recognised and cause few symptoms apart from discomfort. Occasionally an allergic reaction confuses the picture, particularly the large bullae that can occur from bites on the arms and legs. It may be difficult to persuade patients that their recurrent itching spots are simply due to flea bites and the suggestion may be angrily rejected.

Some diseases with skin lesions resulting from insect bites

Condition	Appearance	Organism	Vector
Cutaneous leishmaniasis	Chronic enlarging nodules with ulceration	Leishmania protozoon (*L braziliensis*)	Sand fly
Oriental sore	Ulcerating nodules	Leishmania (*L tropica*)	Sand fly
Kala-azar	Hypopigmented, erythematous, and nodular lesions	Leishmania (*L donovani*)	Insect vectors
Onchocerciasis	Pruritic nodules	Filaria (*Onchocerca volvulus*)	Black fly (Simuliidae)
Typhus, human	Erythematous rash and systemic illness	Rickettsia (*R prowazekii*)	Human louse
Typhus, murine		(*R mooseri*)	Rat flea
Rocky Mountain spotted fever	Maculopapular rash and fever	Rickettsia (*R rickettsii*)	Ticks
Rickettsial pox	Vesicular eruption like chickenpox	Rickettsia (*R akari*)	House mouse, louse
Tick typhus	Necrotic lesions maculopapular rash and fever	Various rickettsias	Ticks
Scrub typhus	Fever, lymphadenopathy, maculopapular rash	Rickettsia (*R tsutsugamushi*)	Mites
Relapsing fever	Widespread maculopapular lesions	*Borrelia recurrentis*	Lice, ticks
Lyme disease	May be annular	*Borrelia burgdorferi*	Ticks, black fly
Yellow fever and dengue	Flushing of face, scarlatiniform rash	Arbovirus	Aedes mosquito

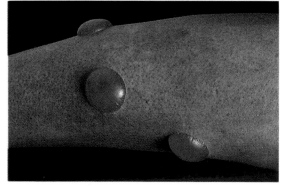

Bullae caused by insect bites.

On the other hand, some patients are convinced that they have an infestation when they do not. Often they will bring small packets containing insects. Examination shows these to be small screws

Insect bites and infestations

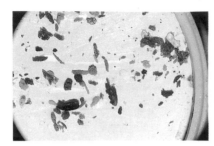

Parasitophobia specimens.

of wool, pickings of keratin, thread, and so on. Sympathy and tact will win patients' confidence; derision and disbelief will merely send them elsewhere for a further medical opinion. Pimozide by mouth may help to dispel the delusion of parasitic infestation (delusional parasitosis).

Some useful points:

(1) Flea bites, including those from cheyletiella mites in dogs and cats, occur in clusters, often in areas of close contact with clothing—for example, around the waist.

(2) Grain mites (pyemotes) and harvest mites (trombicula) can cause severe reactions.

(3) Tick, and possibly mosquito, bites can produce infection with borrelia spirochaetes, causing arthropathy, fever, and a distinctive rash (erythema chronicum migrans)—Lyme disease. The condition responds rapidly to treatment with penicillin. Increasing numbers of cases are being reported in the United Kingdom.

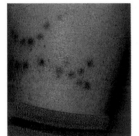
Bites on ankles.

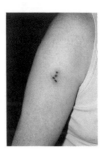
Erythema chronicum migrans.

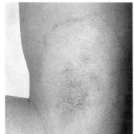

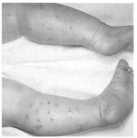
Left: harvest mites; right: papular urticaria.

Papular urticaria

Persistent pruritic (itching) papules in groups on the trunk and legs may be due to bites from fleas, bed bugs, or mites. A seasonal incidence suggests bites from outdoor insects, while recurrence of the papules in a particular house or room suggests infestations with fleas. The term is sometimes used for other causes of itchy skin.

Spider bites

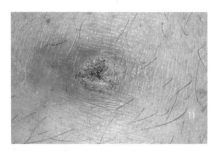
Spider bite (Nigeria).

In Europe spider bites rarely cause problems, but sometimes noxious species arrive in consignments of tropical fruit. The patient shown had been bitten by a spider the day before leaving Nigeria and developed a painful necrotic lesion.

Bites from the European tarantula are painful but otherwise harmless.

In tropical and subtropical countries venomous spiders inject neurotoxins that can be fatal. The "black widow" (*Latrodectus mactans*), "fiddleback," and *Atrax* species of Australia are better known examples. Scorpions cause severe local and systemic symptoms as a result of stings (not bites).

Infestations

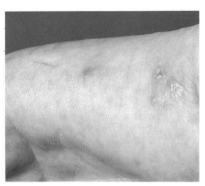
Burrows of scabies.

Scabies

The commonest infestation encountered is scabies, and it is easily missed or misdiagnosed. Scabies is due to a small mite, *Sarcoptes scabiei*. The female mite burrows into the stratum corneum to lay her eggs; the male dies after completing his role of fertilisation, and the developing eggs hatch into larvae within a few days. Intense itching occurs some two weeks later, during which time extensive colonisation may have occurred. The infestation is acquired only by close contact with infected people.

Diagnosis—Finding a burrow—the small (5-10 mm long) ridge, often S shaped—can be difficult as it is often obscured by excoriation from scratching. Without finding a burrow, however, the diagnosis remains uncertain. Isolation of an acarus with a needle or scalpel blade and its demonstration under the microscope convinces the most sceptical patient. Always ask whether there are others in the patient's household and if any of them are itching.

Treatment—Treatment is with gamma benzene hexachloride preparation (Quellada) or 25% benzoyl benzoate emulsion. Important points are:

(1) The patient should wash well: a hot bath was formerly advocated but it is now known that this may increase absorption through the skin.

(2) The lotion should be applied from the neck down, concentrating on affected areas and making sure that the axillae, wrists, ankles, and pubic areas are included. If there is any doubt about the thoroughness of application the process should be repeated in a few days.

(3) Gamma benzene hexachloride (lindane) should not be used for children under 10 or for pregnant women in the first trimester. In such patients crotamiton can be used instead, although this is less effective.

(4) All contacts and members of the patient's household should be treated at the same time.

(5) Residual papules may persist for many weeks. Topical steroids can be used to relieve the itching.

Demodex

Demodex folliculorum is a small mite that inhabits the human hair follicle, the eggs being deposited in the sebaceous gland. It is found on the central area of the face, chest, and neck of adults. It may have a role in the pathogenesis of rosacea, in which it may be found in large numbers. It may be associated with a pustular eruption round the mouth and blepharitis.

Larva migrans

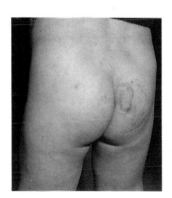

Larva migrans

The boy in the illustration had been on holiday at a coastal town in Kenya and regularly played on a beach frequented by dogs. Two weeks after returning to Britain he started itching on the buttocks and subsequently his parents noticed a linear, raised area that progressed to form a semicircle—a condition known as larva migrans, due to the larvae of the hookworm of dogs and cats, *Ancyclostoma caninum*. The ova are shed in the faeces and in a warm moist environment hatch into larvae that invade "dead end" hosts. They do not develop any further, so systemic disease does not occur. Treatment is either by freezing the advancing end of the lesion with liquid nitrogen or by applying thiabendazole (10%) suspension. Similar lesions in patients returning from tropical countries raises the possibility of larva corneus from strongyloides infestation, myiasis from the larvas of flies, or gnathostomiasis.

Visceral larva migrans caused by *Toxocara canis* and *Ascaris lumbricoides* may produce a transient rash.

Pediculosis (lice)

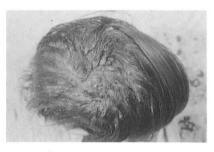

Pediculosis capitis.

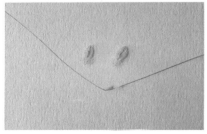

Head lice and nits.

Infestation with lice became less common in the postwar years, but the incidence has recently increased.

There are three areas of the body usually affected by two species of wingless insects—*Pediculus humanus*, infecting the head and body, and *Phthirus pubis*, the pubic louse. The wingless insects feed on blood aspirated at the site of the bite, and each female lays 60-80 encapsulated eggs attached to hairs—"nits" in common parlance.

Head lice are transmitted via combs, brushes, and hats, being more common in girls than boys. The infestation is heaviest behind the ears and over the occiput. If the eyelashes of children are affected this is with "crab lice" (*Phthirus pubis*); it is not pediculosis.

Body lice are less common in western Europe. Transmission is by clothing and bedding, on which both lice and their eggs may be found in the seams. Poor hygiene favours infestation.

Pubic lice infestation occurs world wide and is generally transmitted by sexual contact. Infestation of eyelashes may occur with poor hygiene.

As a result of scratching there may be marked secondary infection that obscures the underlying infestation.

DISEASES OF THE HAIR AND SCALP

The growth cycle

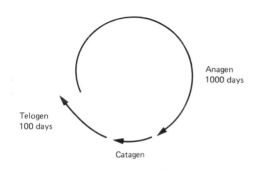

Hair has no vital function in humans, but the lack or excess of it may cause endless misery. Minor "faults" in hair texture, colour, or shape sustain an industry worth billions of pounds a year.

Each hair on the body goes through a cycle of growth independent of its neighbours. The length of each phase of the cycle, as well as its overall length, varies with site and age. For example, in the scalp anagen, the growing phase, averages 1000 days, catagen, when the follicles involute, only a few days, and telogen, a resting state, 100 days. An average scalp contains 100 000 hairs and sheds about 100 "naturally" each day.

There are also long term trends in hair growth: the number of follicles decreases with age, having been maximal at birth.

Telogen effluvium is a common type of diffuse hair loss occurring after pregnancy or after a severe illness. During pregnancy, most hairs move into anagen. After delivery large numbers of these follicles involute (catagen phase) and pass into the resting state, in which no further growth occurs. When anagen starts again, some eight weeks later, the resting hairs are pushed out and lost, causing a temporary diffuse thinning of scalp hair.

Anagen effluvium follows any insult to the hair follicle which cuts down mitosis or weakens the hair shaft. This is the usual way in which drugs cause alopecia.

Hormonal factors—Hair follicles are under hormonal control: androgens and thyroxine are the most important but many others influence them to some extent. All hair is sensitive to androgens, but this is most striking in the secondary sexual hair of the axillae, pubis, and face.

Diseases of the hair fall into three groups:
- Excess hair—hirsutism, hypertrichosis
- Hair loss—alopecia
- Deformity of hair shafts

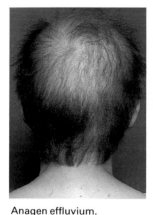

Anagen effluvium.

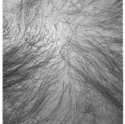

Diffuse alopecia caused by cyclosporin.

Excess of hair

Causes of hirsutism	
● Hereditary, racial	
● Endocrine	
Adrenal	—virilising tumours
	Cushing's syndrome
	adrenal hyperplasia
Ovarian	—virilising tumours
	polycystic ovary
	syndrome
Pituitary	—acromegaly
	hyperprolactinaemia
● Iatrogenic	—anabolic steroids,
	androgens,
	corticosteroids,
	danazol, phenytoin,
	psoralens (in PUVA)

Hirsutism is an excess of coarse secondary sexual hair in a male distribution. *Hypertrichosis* is an excessive growth in any other pattern.

Idiopathic or hereditary causes are by far the most common causes of hirsutism, especially in women from Mediterranean or Arabic countries. The prevalence of hirsutism also increases with age, and even in Caucasians it is common over the age of 60. There is usually a family history and general health is normal. Endocrine investigation is not needed.

Endocrine disease as a cause of hirsutism is rare but should be considered if the hirsutism develops rapidly or if it is associated with obvious virilisation, menstrual disturbances, infertility, or acne. Measurements of serum testosterone and urinary 17-oxosteroid concentrations are useful screening tests.

Treatment—The treatment of idiopathic hirsutism includes:

(*a*) depilatory creams or shaving; there is no evidence that these lead to increased growth or pigmentation of the hair;

(*b*) electrolysis and diathermy;

(*c*) in severe cases, the antiandrogen cyproterone, but this should be used only under specialist supervision.

Excess hair in men is seldom a problem.

Hypertrichosis is rare and usually has an obvious cause. Treatment is directed to any underlying problem.

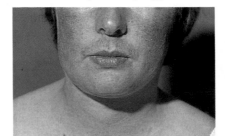

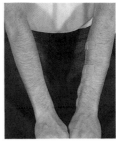

Hirsuties due to virilising tumour.

Hypertrichosis caused by minoxidil.

Causes of hypertrichosis
- Congenital (rare)
- Acquired—porphyria
  hyperthyroidism
  anorexia nervosa
  some developmental defects
  eg Hurler's syndrome
  tumours (hypertrichosis
  lanuginosa)
  drugs (diazoxide, minoxidil,
  cyclosporin)

Alopecia

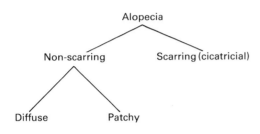

Causes of diffuse non-scarring alopecia
- Androgenetic
  alopecia —male pattern
  —female pattern
- Endocrine —thyroid disease
  (hypothyroidism and
  hyperthyroidism)
  —hypopituitarism
  —diabetes mellitus
- Stress —postpartum
  —postoperative } telogen effluvium
  —postfebrile
- Drugs —cytotoxics
  —anticoagulants
  —antithyroid } anagen effluvium
  agents
  —cyclosporin
- Erythrodermic skin
  disease —psoriasis
  —eczema
  —lymphoma
- Deficiency
  states —protein malnutrition
  —iron deficiency

Alopecia can be classified into scarring or non-scarring types and the non-scarring types into diffuse or patchy. Scarring alopecia is usually associated with a concurrent skin disease, whereas in non-scarring alopecia the primary process affects the hair follicle.

Destruction of the hair follicle leads to plugging, atrophy (a fine and wrinkled appearance), and loss of the normally visible follicular orifices. The microscopic examination of plucked hairs may be useful, as may be a skin biopsy.

Remember that alopecia may reflect an underlying systemic disease or be a local manifestation of a generalised skin disease. A full history and examination are essential.

Non-scarring alopecia

Androgenetic alopecia (common baldness) in men, starts with frontotemporal thinning and then loss from the crown. These bald areas gradually become confluent, leaving only a rim of hair round the edge of the scalp. In women the pattern is more often diffuse and starts later and only rarely does the pattern resemble that of men. Testosterone is responsible but measuring serum concentrations is unhelpful because the underlying cause is hypersensitivity of the hair follicles to normal circulating concentrations of the hormone.

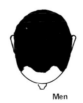   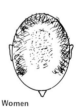

Men

Women

Treatment is ineffective. The value of topical minoxidil is limited. Meanwhile the "virility" theory (in men) may help some.

In hypothyroidism the hair is coarse, dry, and thin. Often the first indication is that the hair does not take a perm as it should.

Telogen and anagen effluvium have been discussed earlier.

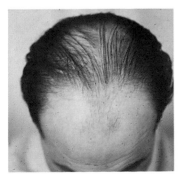

Male pattern baldness.

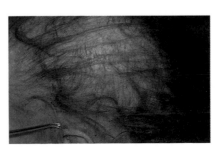

Diffuse alopecia caused by erythrodermic psoriasis.

Diseases of the hair and scalp

Patchy alopecia

Alopecia areata accounts for 2% of dermatological referrals in the United Kingdom. The peak incidence is in early adulthood. It is associated with autoimmune disease and with atopy. There is evidence of an immunological attack on the hair follicle.

There are usually no other signs apart from the alopecia and, sometimes, a slight erythema. The typical exclamation mark hairs are helpful in diagnosis.

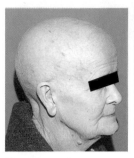
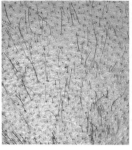
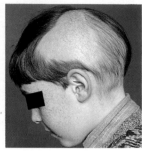

Alopecia totalis.

Alopecia areata, showing exclamation mark hairs.

Alopecia areata.

The prognosis is unpredictable; often the hairs regrow after a few weeks. However, a gradual loss of scalp hair may lead to total alopecia. In severe cases the body hair may also be lost. Rapid evolution, loss of hair from the eyebrows, alopecia totalis, or loss of occipital hair are poor prognostic factors.

Treatment is disappointing. The injection of intralesional triamcinolone may induce a temporary regrowth and help psychologically. Permanent regrowth may not be achieved.

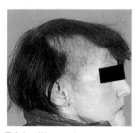
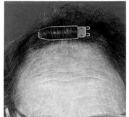

Trichotillomania.

Traction alopecia.

Trichotillomania is the constant plucking of hair by a patient who may be psychologically disturbed. The unusual pattern and the mental state of the patient usually makes the diagnosis straightforward. Treatment is often unsuccessful.

Traction alopecia is caused by an abnormal tug on the hair shafts from hairdressing accessories, such as tight rollers.

Scarring (cicatricial) alopecia

Hair follicles can be destroyed in several ways (see box). Acute inflammation is usually of infective origin. In preantibiotic days the moth eaten alopecia of syphilis was common.

Lupus erythematosus may affect the scalp in both its discoid and systemic forms. In the discoid type a heavy scale is seen with plugging of the hair follicles. A similar picture occurs in lichen planus, and the rash of lichen planus may be seen more typically elsewhere. Morphoea (localised scleroderma) may affect the scalp, the *en coup de sabre* pattern being one variant.

A slowly extending area of alopecia may suggest a cicatricial basal cell carcinoma.

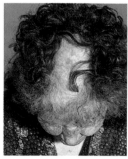
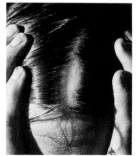

Systemic lupus erythematosus.

En coup de sabre.

The treatment of scarring alopecia must be swift and directed at its underlying cause. Once scarring is present alopecia is irreversible. Potent topical steroids help in lupus erythematosus and lichen planus.

Hair shaft defects

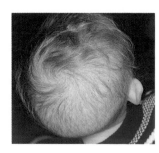
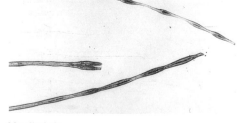

Monilethrix.

Defects of the hair shaft are rare disorders leading to weakness or breaking of the hairs. Often they are inherited. The hairs may have a distinctive appearance, most evident on microscopy.

Examples of these defects include monilethrix and pili torti. Treatment is unsatisfactory.

Diseases of the scalp

The scalp is the site of predilection for several skin diseases, which are listed in the box, but seldom is the scalp the only site affected. Some have been dealt with under scarring alopecia and others in previous chapters.

Pityriasis capitis is the commonest skin complaint after acne, and indeed a mild dandruff is physiological. Reactions to *Pityrosporum ovale*, a normal yeast commensal, may play a part in its pathogenesis. Occasionally masses of sticky scale may heap up, matting adjacent hairs together. This picture is known as *pityriasis amiantacea*. A similar appearance may be seen in scalp psoriasis. The treatment of pityriasis capitis includes tar and salicylic acid preparations, and shampoos containing selenium or zinc pyrithione.

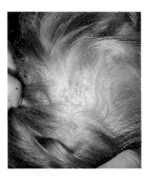
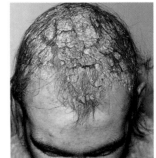

Left: tinea capitis; right: pityriasis amiantacea.

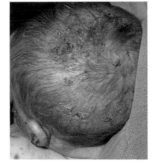
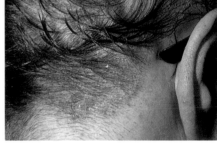

Atopic eczema.

Contact eczema, hair dye.

DISEASES OF THE NAILS

Nail fold · Nail plate · Nail bed · Nail matrix

Nails are a protective cover for the ends of the fingers and toes which also help to increase tactile sensitivity by exerting counterpressure over the distal pulp.

The nail consists of a nail plate resting on the nail bed, which grows out from a nail matrix.

Fingernails grow about 1 cm in three months and toenails at about a third of this rate. Growth is slower in the non-dominant hand and in old age.

Examination and surface changes

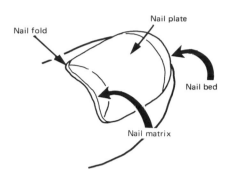

Pits

Psoriasis
Alopecia
Hand dermatitis

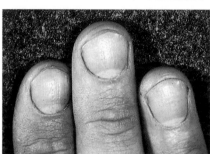

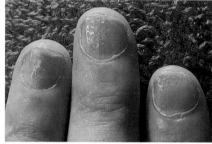

Horizontal ridging

Beau's lines
Previous systemic illness
Hand dermatitis

Longitudinal ridges

Single
Pressure effect
Multiple
Lichen planus
Alopecia areata
Psoriasis
Darier's disease

A thorough relevant history is essential. Particular attention should be paid to past skin conditions because a previous episode of hand dermatitis may have settled leaving perplexing nail changes. A family history of psoriasis may explain nail changes in the absence of any other such signs. Occupation may also be relevant.

The nails should always be examined in adequate light, and all the fingernails and toenails should be inspected. Particular attention should be paid to the symmetry of the changes. For example, onychomycosis and psoriasis may cause similar changes, but psoriasis is commonly symmetrical while onychomycosis is often not.

Other signs of skin disease should be carefully looked for. Psoriasis can cause severe nail changes with no other skin lesions, but a thorough examination may show a small patch of psoriasis periumbilically or perianally.

An assessment should then be made of which parts of the nail are affected. Are the changes in the surface texture of the nail, the nail plate itself, the nail bed, or the surrounding soft tissues?

Pits are small punctate depressions in the nail plate. They vary considerably in size and may be regular or irregular. They occur commonly in psoriasis, usually irregularly distributed, and in alopecia areata, when they may be very regular. They are less commonly associated with hand dermatitis.

Horizontal ridging is usually seen in the form of Beau's line. This is usually a single horizontal depression that progresses distally with nail growth and indicates a previous episode of illness. Multiple small horizontal ridges may occur with hand dermatitis or any inflammatory condition affecting the soft tissues around the nail.

Longitudinal ridges—Single longitudinal ridges may be caused by pressure from tumours, either benign or malignant, in the proximal nail fold. These may progress to a true split in the nail.

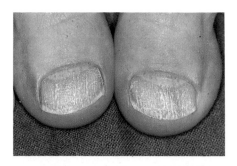

Trachyonychia

Lichen planus
Psoriasis
Alopecia areata

Multiple longitudinal ridges of varying size are a feature of lichen planus, psoriasis, alopecia areata, and Darier's disease. When lichen planus is suspected the buccal mucosal membrane should always be examined for lesions.

Trachyonychia is roughness of the nails, so that they feel like fine sandpaper. This change is usually symmetrical and can occur in lichen planus, psoriasis, and alopecia areata.

Changes in the nail plate

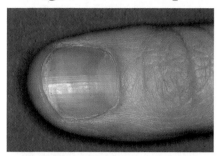

Thickening

Psoriasis
Onychomycosis
Pachyonychia congenita

Thickening or hypertrophy of the nail plate is most commonly seen with psoriasis and onychomycosis. The changes are often asymmetrical. The presence of other nail changes due to psoriasis (such as pitting and onycholysis) should be sought if there are no other skin signs of psoriasis. Nail clippings may need to be taken for microscopy and culture to exclude fungal infection. More rarely the changes may affect all the nails as in pachyonychia congenita.

Lamellar splitting of the nail plate occurs distally and horizontally and is caused by exogenous factors, particularly repeated immersion in water.

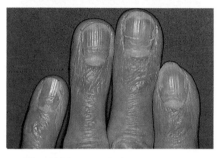

Lamellar splitting
Trauma

Onychomadesis is complete shedding of the nail and can occur in any severe illness which results in sudden stopping of nail growth. The nail plate continues to move distally and is shed when it loses its adhesion to underlying tissues. This change may rarely occur with lichen planus. Shedding may be seen with any condition which can cause severe onycholysis.

Shedding—
onychomadesis

Systemic illness
Lichen planus

Detachment—
onycholysis

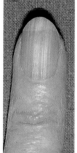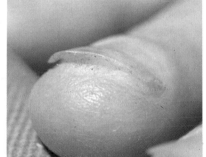

Psoriasis
Onychomycosis
Trauma
Thyrotoxicosis

Onycholysis is detachment of the nail from its bed. The main difference from onychomadesis is that it usually, but not always, begins distally or laterally, causing a subungual space which fills with air, giving that area of the nail a whitish grey discoloration. It is most commonly seen in psoriasis but can occur in onychomycosis, thyrotoxicosis, and trauma. It may become extensive, enough to cause nail loss, through loosening of the nail plate.

Onychogryphosis is thickening of the nail, probably due to repeated trauma. It commonly affects the nails of both great toes but may affect other toes as well.

Subungual hyperkeratosis is due to hyperplasia of the epidermis underlying the nail plate and occurs either distally or throughout the nail. It is usually seen in psoriasis and hand dermatitis.

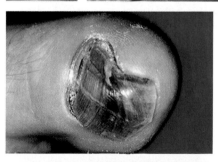

Thickening—
onychogryphosis

Trauma

Colour changes in the nail plate—Apparent changes in colour may be caused by changes in the nail bed. Cyanosis may make the nails look blue. Actual discoloration of the nail plate can be due to endogenous or exogenous factors. *Exogenous* factors include occupational exposure to dyes or other materials. Infection with pseudomonas may colour the nail green and topical treatment may stain the nail plate—for example, potassium permanganate soaks stain it brown. Prolonged application of nail varnish may also make nails brown. *Endogenous* causes of discoloration include a wide variety of drugs and systemic illnesses.

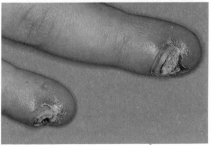

Subungual
hyperkeratosis

Psoriasis
Hand dermatitis

Diseases of the nails

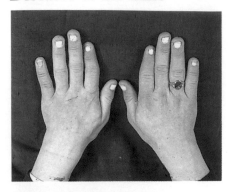

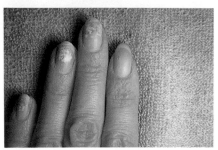

Leukonychia

True
Onychomycosis
Trauma

Apparent
Anaemia
Hypoproteinaemia

Colour changes

Exogenous
Occupational
Pseudomonas infection
Topical treatment

Endogenous
Drugs, eg
   Tetracyclines—yellow
   Antimalarials—blue
   Chlorpromazine—brown
Systemic illness, eg
   Jaundice—yellow
   Cirrhosis—white
   Adrenal insufficiency—
    brown

Koilonychia

Iron deficiency

Pigmented streaks

Malignant melanoma

Normal in pigmented skin
Melanocytic naevi
Lentigo
Addison's disease

Koilonychia is a spoon shaped deformity of the nail plate, which may also be thinned. The changes may be asymmetrical. The fingers are usually more affected than the toes. It is most characteristically seen in association with iron deficiency anaemia but may be idiopathic.

Leukonychia or whiteness of the nails is said to be true when it affects the nail plate and apparent when it affects the subungual tissues. Complete whiteness of the nail is rare, but isolated total leukonychia is seen with fungal infections. The only common form of true leukonychia is the punctate form, which occurs as small white spots 1-3 mm in diameter, singly or in groups. This probably relates to episodes of trauma to the nail matrix. Apparent leukonychia is seen in anaemia and hypoproteinaemia.

Pigmented streaks—Longitudinal pigmented streaks may be multiple in pigmented skin and are a normal finding. Their presence in white people, particularly if of recent onset, raises the possibility of a malignant melanoma of the nail. These may or may not produce dystrophic changes in the nail plate. Twenty five per cent of subungual melanomas are amelanotic. Other causes of pigmented streaks include conditions such as a lentigo, as well as benign melanocytic naevi. Similar changes may be seen in Addison's disease.

Around the nail: soft tissue changes

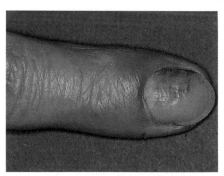

Paronychia

Acute
Trauma

Chronic
Trauma
Water

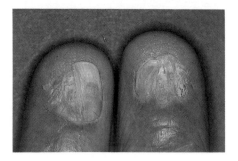

Pterygium formation

Circulatory disorders
Lichen planus

Paronychia is probably the commonest of nail complaints. When it occurs acutely it usually begins at the side of the nail with redness and swelling. Pus may collect which requires drainage. The commonest infecting organisms are staphylococci and less commonly β haemolytic streptococci. Correct antibiotic therapy is essential.

The condition may present as a more chronic problem characterised by loss of the cuticle over all or part of the nail with thickening of the nail fold and variable inflammation.

Acute paronychia usually affects only one nail, whereas chronic paronychias may affect several. The cause may also be different. Acute paronychia is often related to minor trauma whereas the chronic state usually results from repeated immersion in water, and *Candida albicans* can be isolated in many cases.

Pterygium formation—The cuticle appears to grow out over the nail with loss of the proximal nail fold. Initially this may appear to split the nail but can progress to complete nail loss. It is due to a scarring loss of the nail matrix and is seen in conditions characterised by impairment of the circulation and occasionally in lichen planus.

Treatment of nail disorders

Treatment of chronic paronychia

Keep hands as dry as possible

Treat episodes of inflammation with oral antibiotics

Long term application of ointment containing nystatin or antiseptic paint, eg gentian violet

---

Few specific treatments are successful for nail disorders, except for fungal infections, which are usually treated with oral griseofulvin. Griseofulvin may need to be given for more than a year and even then may not produce complete clearance, particularly of the toenails. Tablets should be taken with food. Like many treatments, griseofulvin should not be given in pregnancy. Side effects commonly consist of gastrointestinal disturbances and less commonly headaches, photosensitivity, and allergic reactions. Ketoconazole is an alternative and it needs to be given for the same length of time. Liver toxicity has been reported and regular monitoring is necessary.

Other nail dystrophies

Psoriatic nail changes may improve if the general state of the skin improves. Potent topical steroids applied locally can produce some improvement but relapse is frequent.

Local eczematous disease—Changes related to a local eczematous process will gradually improve if the local skin remains clear.

Non-scarring lichen planus improves spontaneously. Progressive scarring may be helped by oral steroids. The nail changes of alopecia areata may persist after the hair loss has recovered. Treatment is unhelpful.

Local trauma—Problems related to local trauma, particularly chronic paronychia, lamellar splitting, and onycholysis, will improve if the underlying factors can be removed.

Further reading

Samman PD. *The nails in disease*. 3rd ed. London: Heinemann, 1978.
Baran R, Dawber RPR. *Diseases of the nail and their management*. Oxford: Blackwell Scientific, 1984.

LUMPS AND BUMPS

The skin is a common site for neoplastic lesions, but most invade only locally and with treatment usually do not pose any threat to the life of the patient. The exception is malignant melanoma, which is dealt with in the next chapter. This is a rare tumour with a high mortality, and recent publicity campaigns have been aimed at preventing the tragedy of fatal metastases from a neglected melanoma.

As a result a large number of patients are being seen with pigmented skin lesions and nodules, only a very few of which are neoplastic. The question is how to distinguish the benign, the malignant, and the possibly malignant. The following guidelines may help in deciding whether the lesion can be safely left or should be treated.

A correlation of the clinical and pathological features is helpful in making a confident diagnosis of the more common tumours.

Seborrhoeic warts

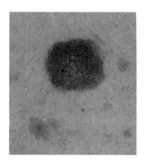 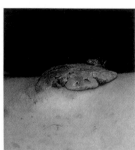

Seborrhoeic warts come in various shapes, sizes, and colours. When deeply pigmented, inflamed, or growing they may appear to have the features of a malignant lesion, but the following features are characteristic.
● Well defined edge
● Warty, papillary surface—often with keratin plugs
● Raised above surrounding skin to give a "stuck on" appearance.
Individual lesions vary considerably in size, but are usually 0·5-3 cm in diameter. Protruberant and pedunculated lesions occur. Solitary lesions are commonly seen on the face and neck but more numerous, large lesions tend to occur on the trunk. They become more common with increasing age.

Basal cell carcinoma

In contrast, the early basal cell carcinoma—or rodent ulcer—presents as a firm nodule, clearly growing within the skin and below it, rather than on the surface. The colour varies from that of normal skin to dark brown or black, but there is commonly a "pearly" translucent quality. As its name implies, the tumour is composed of masses of dividing basal cells that have lost the capacity to differentiate any further. As a result no epidermis is formed over

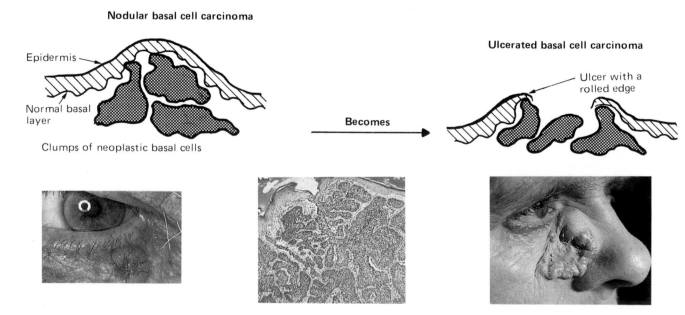

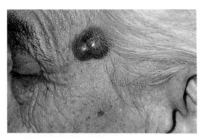
Cystic basal cell carcinoma.

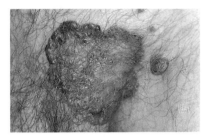
Superficial basal cell carcinoma.

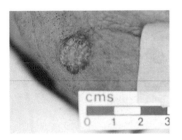
Pigmented basal cell carcinoma.

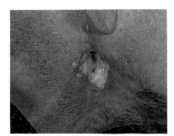
Neglected basal cell carcinoma (rodent ulcer).

the tumour and the surface breaks down to form an ulcer, the residual edges of the nodule forming the characteristic "rolled edge." Once the basal cells have invaded the deeper tissues the rolled edge disappears.

Variants

Variants of the usual pattern can cause problems in diagnosis. *Cystic* basal cell carcinomas occur and those that show differentiation towards hair follicles or sweat glands may have a less typical appearance. *Pigmented* lesions can resemble melanoma. The *superficial spreading* type may be confused with a patch of eczema. This usually occurs on the trunk, does not itch, and shows a gradual but inexorable increase in size. A firm "whipcord" edge may be present.

Treatment

Various methods of destroying tumour tissue are used and the results are similar for radiotherapy and surgical excision.
(1) Ulcerated lesions may invade tissue planes, blood vessels, and nerves more extensively than is clinically apparent.
(2) Although modern techniques of radiotherapy result in minimal scarring and atrophy these may cause problems near the eye.
(3) Basal cell carcinomas in skin creases, such as the nasolabial fold, tend to ulcerate and are hard to excise adequately.
(4) Surgical excision has the advantage that should the lesion recur radiotherapy is available to treat it, whereas it is not desirable to treat recurrences after radiotherapy with further irradiation.

Squamous cell carcinoma

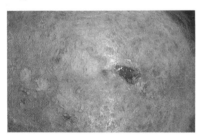

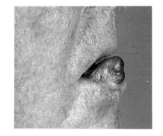

Squamous cell carcinoma

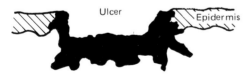
Squamous neoplastic cells

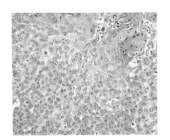

Squamous cell carcinoma represents proliferation of the epidermal keratinocytes in a deranged manner—with a variable degree of differentiation into epidermal cells that may show individual cell keratinisation and "pearls" of keratin. In other tumours bizarre cells with mitoses, cells with clear cytoplasm, or spindle cells may be seen.

This type of cancer often develops at a site of previous damage to the skin—for example, from sunlight or chemical damage. The first change clinically is a thickening of the skin with scaling or hyperkeratosis of the surfaces. The more differentiated tumours often have a warty, keratotic crust while others may be nodular. The edge is poorly defined. There may be associated dilated, telangiectatic blood vessels. The original hard, disc like lesion becomes nodular and ulcerates with strands of tumour cells invading the deeper tissue. The thick warty crust, often found elsewhere, may be absent from lesions on the lip, buccal mucosa, and penis.

These histological changes complement the clinical appearance and are clearly different from those of basal cell carcinoma.

Treatment—Small lesions should be excised as a rule, making sure that the palpable edge of the tumour is included, with a 3-5 mm margin. Radiotherapy is effective but fragile scars may be a disadvantage on the hand. Cryotherapy or topical fluorouracil can be used for histologically confirmed, superficial lesions and also for solar keratoses.

Lumps and bumps
Solar keratoses

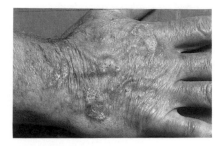

Squamous cell carcinoma may develop in solar keratoses, which show thickening of the epidermis and abnormal keratinocytes. They occur on sites exposed to the sun and are more common on those who have worked out of doors or sunbathed excessively. They can be regarded as squamous cell carcinomas grade 1/2 but do not necessarily progress to a dysplastic carcinoma. They also develop on the lips, particularly of pipe smokers.

The clinical appearance varies from a simple rough area of skin to a keratotic lesion with marked inflammation. The edge and surface are irregular.

Treatment with cryotherapy, using liquid nitrogen or carbon dioxide, repeated if necessary, is usually effective.

Other conditions

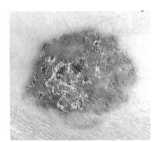

Bowen's disease.

Bowen's disease is characterised by a well defined, erythematous macule with little induration and slight crusting. It is a condition of the middle aged and elderly, occurring commonly on the trunk and limbs. It is an intraepidermal carcinoma, which has been reported to follow the ingestion of arsenic in "tonics" taken in years gone by or exposure to sheep dip, weedkiller, or industrial processes. After many years florid carcinoma may develop with invasion of deeper tissues. It may be confused with a patch of eczema or superficial basal cell carcinoma. Lesions on covered areas may be associated with underlying malignancy. Erythroplasia of Queyrat is a similar process occurring on the glans penis or prepuce.

Paget's disease of the nipple presents with unilateral non-specific erythematous changes on the aureola and nipple, spreading to the surrounding skin. The cause is an underlying adenocarcinoma of the ducts. It should be considered in any patient with eczematous changes of one breast that fail to respond to simple treatment. Extramammary lesions occur.

Keratoacanthoma is a rapidly growing fleshy nodule that develops a hard keratotic centre. Healing occurs with some scarring. Although benign, it may recur after being removed with curette and cautery, particularly from the face, and is best excised.

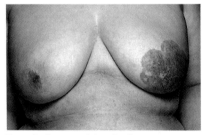

Paget's disease of the nipple.

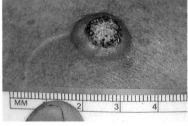

Keratoacanthoma.

Benign tumours

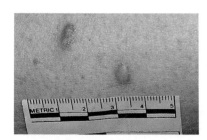

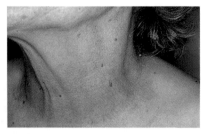

Dermatofibroma (top left), skin tags (above), and syringoma (left).

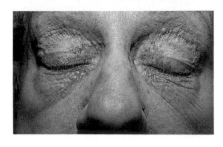

Derma tofibroma—This is a simple, discrete firm nodule, arising in the dermis at the site of an insect bite or other trivial injury. Often there is a brown or red vascular lesion initially which then becomes fibrotic—a sclerosing haemangioma. The histiocytoma is similar but composed of histiocytes.

Skin tags may be pigmented but rarely cause any diagnostic problems unless inflamed. Some are in fact pedunculated seborrhoeic warts and others simple papillomas (fibroepithelial polyps).

Other benign tumours

A wide variety of tumours may develop from the hair follicle and sebaceous, exocrine (sweat), and apocrine glands. The more common include *syringomas* slowly growing, small, multiple nodules on the face of eccrine gland origin.

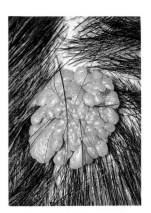

Naevus sebaceous.

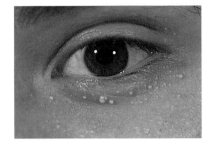

Verrucous epidermal naevus.

Naevus sebaceous is warty, well defined, varying in size from a small nodule to one several centimetres in diameter. Lesions occur in the scalp of children, may be present at birth, and gradually increase in size. They may proliferate or develop into a basal cell carcinoma in adult life and they are therefore best removed.

Verrucous epidermal naevi are probably a variant, found on the trunk and limbs.

Cysts

The familiar *epidermoid cyst*—also known as sebaceous cyst or wen—occurs as a soft, well defined, mobile swelling usually on the face, neck, shoulder, and chest. It is not derived from sebaceous glands but contains keratin produced by the lining wall.

Pilar cysts on the scalp are similar lesions derived from hair follicles.

Milia are small keratin cysts consisting of small white papules found on the cheek and eyelids.

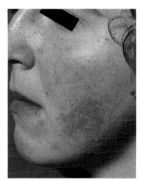

Epidermoid cyst.

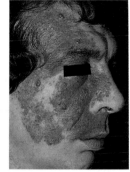

Milia.

Vascular lesions

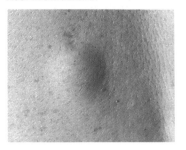

Naevus flammeus.

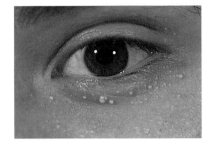

Sturge-Weber syndrome.

The more common vascular naevi are mentioned.

The port wine stain, or naevus flammeus, presents at birth as a flat red lesion, usually on the face, neck, or upper trunk. There is usually a sharp midline border on the more common unilateral lesions. In time the affected area becomes raised and thickened because of proliferation of vascular and connective tissue. If the area supplied by the ophthalmic or maxillary divisions of the trigeminal nerve is affected there may be associated angiomas of the underlying meninges with epilepsy —Sturge-Weber syndrome. Lesions of the limb may be associated with arteriovenous fistulae.

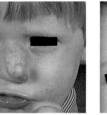

Cavernous angioma.

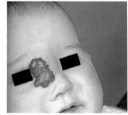

Cavernous angioma—strawberry naevi—appear in the first few weeks of life or at birth. A soft vascular swelling is found, most commonly on the head and neck. The lesions resolve spontaneously in time and do not require treatment.

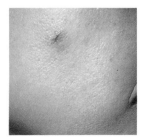

Spider naevi.

Pyogenic granuloma.

Spider naevus consist of a central vascular papule with fine lines radiating from it. They are more common in children and women. Large numbers in a man raise the possibility of liver disease.

Campbell de Morgan spots are discrete red papules 1-5 mm in diameter. They are more common on the trunk.

Pyogenic granuloma is a lesion that contains no pus but is in fact vascular and grows rapidly.

It may arise at the site of trauma. Distinction from amelanotic melanoma is important.

BLACK SPOTS IN THE SKIN

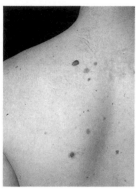

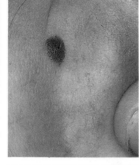

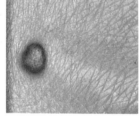

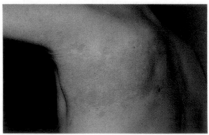

Benign pigmented naevi.

Any dark lesion of the skin may be a cause for concern, sometimes regarded by the patient with the same dread as Long John Silver's "black spot" in *Treasure Island*—a sign of imminent demise. However, the vast majority of pigmented lesions are entirely harmless naevi.

Most of us acquire "moles" or pigmented naevi in childhood and early adult life. These fade gradually in old age. They are composed of cells derived from melanocytes of the epidermal basal layer, with a variable amount of connective tissue as well.

The clinical appearance varies from a flat pigmented macule (*melanocytic naevus*) to a protruberant nodule bearing hair (*compound naevus*) with variable proportions of pigmented naevus cells and connective tissue. Malignant change is very rare. The exception is found in patients with the *uncommon dysplastic naevus syndrome*, in which multiple naevi develop during adolescence, many of which show the features of malignant change outlined below.

Benign naevi

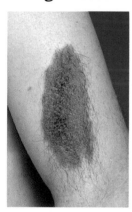

Congenital hairy naevus.

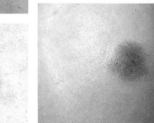

Blue naevus.

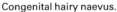

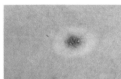

Halo naevus.

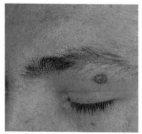

Spitz naevus.

Congenital pigmented naevi present at, or soon after, birth as dark hairy lesions, which become more protruberant in time. There is a tendency to malignant change. The very large lesions covering much of the trunk or buttocks (bathing trunk naevi) present considerable problems in their removal.

Other benign pigmented naevi include the following.

The blue naevus, presenting as a stable, deep blue, dermal lesion in children and young adults.

The *Spitz naevus* is a fleshy pink papule in children—composed of large spindle cells and epithelial cells in "nests." It is benign and the old name of jevenile melanoma should be abandoned.

A *halo naevus* consists of a central melanocytic naevi with a depigmented halo, caused by an autoimmune reaction. The central naevus gradually involutes. Vitiligo may be present elsewhere.

Becker's naevus consist of a faintly pigmented area, often on the upper trunk or shoulder with an increase in hair density. It is benign.

Freckles or ephelides are small (less than 0·5 cm) pigmented macules that occur on exposure to sunlight in fair skinned people and fade during the winter.

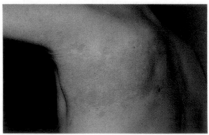

Becker's naevus.

Malignant melanomas

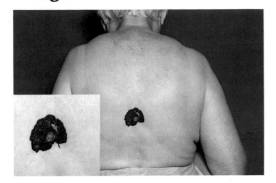

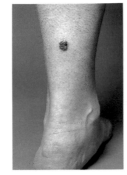

Melanoma is an invasive malignant tumour of melanocytes. Most cases occur in adults over the age of 30 with fair complexions. The condition is also more common in women, in whom melanomas often occur on the lower leg. The table shows the criteria for suspecting malignant changes in pigmented lesions. Any change in a skin lesion is a reason to assess the lesion carefully, and if more than two of the features in the table are present it is generally accepted that the patient should be referred for a specialist opinion.

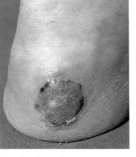

Dysplastic melanoma.

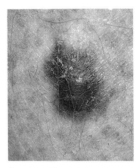

Amelanotic melanoma.

Criteria for suspecting malignant changes in pigmented lesions

(1) *Itching*—Normally a mole does not itch but a melanoma may. Irritated seborrhoeic warts also itch.

(2) *Inflammation* is, of course, a feature of irritated or infected benign lesions, but it occurs in melanoma spontaneously, particularly in the early stages.

(3) *Size*—Apart from congenital pigmented naevi, most benign moles are less than 1 cm in diameter. Any lesion over 0·5 cm should be carefully checked.

(4) *Growth*—Benign pigmented naevi continue to appear in adolescents and young adults. Any mole increasing in size in an adult over the age of 30 may be a melanoma.

(5) *Shape*—Moles usually have a symmetrical, even outline, any indentations being quite regular, but melanomas usually have an irregular edge with one part advancing more than the others.

(6) *Colour*—Variation in colour of benign moles is even but a melanoma may be intensely black or show irregular coloration varying from white to slate blue, with all shades of black and brown. Inflammation may give a red colour as well. The "amelanotic" melanoma shows little or no pigmentation.

(7) *Surface breakdown* with bleeding and crusting occurs in an actively growing melanoma.

If more than two of these features are present refer the patient for a specialist opinion

A simple summary:
A—Asymmetry of the lesion
B—irregularity of the border
C—variations in colour
D—Diameter larger than 0·5 cm

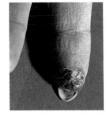

Nodule developing in superficial spreading melanoma.

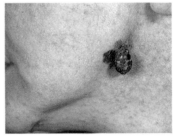

Superficial spreading melanoma.

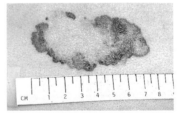

Acral melanoma.

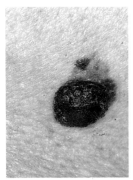

Nodular melanoma.

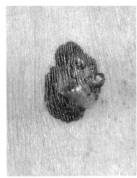

Superficial melanoma with nodules.

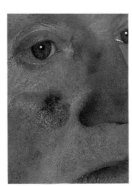

Lentigo maligna.

The commonest clinical type is a spreading lesion with irregular surface and pigmentation.

The nodular variety is less common but grows more rapidly and is more likely to be confused with benign moles.

Highly dysplastic lesions may lose the capacity to produce pigment, resulting in an *amelanotic melanoma*.

The even flat brown lentigo on the face of elderly patients grows slowly over the years. *Lentigo maligna melanoma* is a flat, superficial low grade melanoma. However, a nodular raised portion indicates the development of more rapidly growing invasive melanoma and the need for urgent treatment.

Black spots in the skin

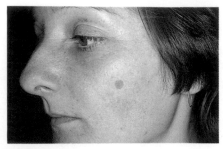

Benign lentigo.

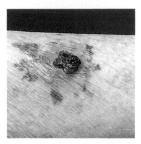

Nodular melanoma
in a lentigo.

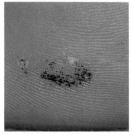

Talon noir.

Acral melanoma occurs on the soles and palms and under the nails (subungual melanoma). Benign pigmented naevi may also occur in these sites, but the seven points in the table will help to differentiate them. *Talon noir*, due to haemorrhage from trauma—for example, playing squash—may cause much concern but the distinct blood filled papillae seen on paring the lesion make the diagnosis plain.

The prognosis of malignant melanoma is related to the depth of invasion. Superficial lesions with a tumour thickness of less than 1 mm have a good prognosis if removed early (80-90% survival at five years). Histologically, the thickness of the tumour is measured from the granular layer (Breslow thickness). Deeper invasion carries a poor prognosis (only 40-50% survival for a tumour deeper than 3 mm).

It is therefore very important to remove any malignant melanoma while it is in the superficial stage, if possible.

PRACTICAL PROCEDURES

Skin biopsy

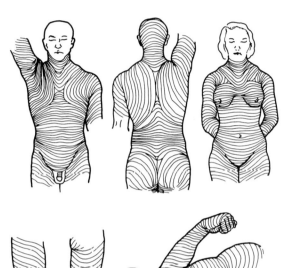

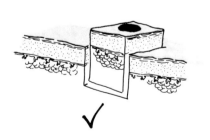

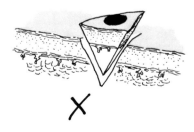

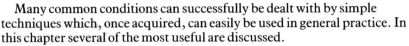

Many common conditions can successfully be dealt with by simple techniques which, once acquired, can easily be used in general practice. In this chapter several of the most useful are discussed.

Skin biopsy is used to establish a diagnosis (incisional) or to remove a lesion (excisional). In both cases the incision should be elliptical and should run parallel to the skin wrinkle lines.

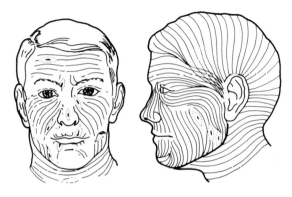

As a rule of thumb the long axis of the wound should be about three times as long as its short axis. The apical angle should be no more than 30°.

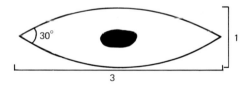

Procedure

(1) Explain the procedure to the patient, warning about the scar that will result from it. This may be slight on the face but more prominent in areas susceptible to keloid formation, such as the sternum, shoulders, and upper outer arms.

(2) Establish that the patient is not allergic to local anaesthetics.

(3) Obtain consent.

(4) Mark out the planned incision with sterile gentian violet before injecting the local anaesthetic.

(5) Anaesthetise with 1-2% plain lignocaine. Lignocaine-adrenaline combinations, though they help to reduce bleeding, should not be used on the extremities. The mild discomfort of the injection may be lessened by injecting very slowly and avoiding lignocaine-adrenaline mixtures.

(6) A number 15 blade is used, cutting at 90° to the skin surface. Wedge shaped incisions heal poorly, as illustrated.

(7) A skin hook may be used to lift one end of the specimen to release its underside. Forceps crush specimens and cause pathological artefacts.

(8) Removal of sutures—from the face at 4-5 days, from the trunk at 7 days, and from the leg at 10 days.

(9) Elevation and compression bandaging are advisable when removing lesions from the lower leg.

Practical procedures

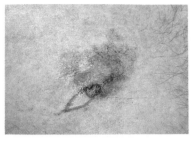

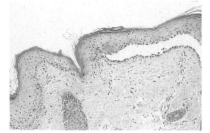

Incisional biopsy—Always include the boundary of the normal-abnormal area in an incisional biopsy specimen, which must be at least 1 cm long and deep enough to include subcutaneous tissue.

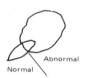
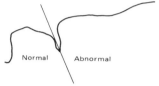

Excisional biopsy—There are several points to remember when removing a lesion.

(1) Allow for an adequate zone of clearance, especially when excising pigmented or neoplastic lesions. A 2·5-5 mm margin is usually sufficient. Partial removal must be avoided.

(2) Place specimens, dermal side down, on a small square of filter paper, to avoid curling, and then immerse them in formalin.

(3) Mark clearly on the specimen container the patient's name and the date of biopsy.

(4) Record on the pathology form the site of biopsy, a description of the lesion and a note of its duration, the clinical history, and the clinical diagnosis.

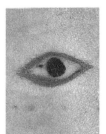
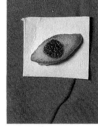
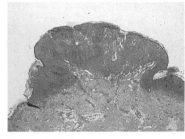

Clinical. Surgical. Histopathological.

Curettage

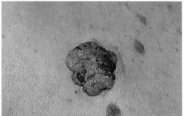
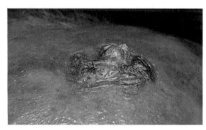

Curettage is ideal for benign epidermal lesions, such as seborrhoeic and actinic keratoses or viral warts.

If well localised on the face, trunk, and limbs superficial or small nodulocystic basal cell carcinomas may be treated by curettage if they have clearcut borders and a firm base. Such specimens must be sent for histological confirmation and the scars reviewed regularly.

Seborrhoeic keratosis. Actinic keratosis.

Procedure

(1) Anaesthetise site.

(2) Stretch the skin on either side of the lesion.

(3) Apply the lip of the curette to the edge of the lesion, as illustrated.

(4) Use a rapid downward scooping action, working around the lesion towards its centre.

(5) Curette down to the dermis, identifiable by its scratchy, sandpaper-like consistency.

(6) Use light cautery, sweeping across the base of the lesion, and pay particular attention to bleeding points. Necrotic tissue produced by excessive cautery impairs wound healing: simple pressure to control bleeding is preferable to this.

(7) Repeat the whole procedure if treating a basal cell carcinoma.

(8) Cover with a dry dressing on the trunk: leave facial lesions exposed. Tell the patient that a scab will form and drop off in about 10 days.

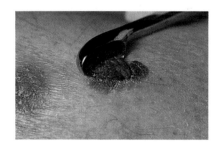

Cryotherapy

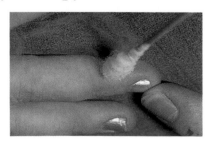

Cryotherapy is used increasingly to treat many dermatological conditions in hospital and general practice. Suitable conditions include (*a*) viral warts and molluscum contagiosum; (*b*) keratoses, both seborrhoeic and actinic; and (*c*) biopsy proved Bowen's disease.

A liquid nitrogen spray may be used but equally good results can be obtained with a cottonwool dipstick method. The best results are then achieved by "rolling your own." After immersing the cottonwool bud in liquid nitrogen apply it firmly to the lesion.

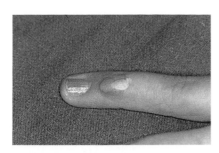

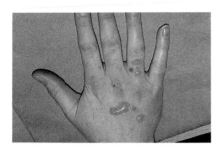

Wait until a thin "halo" of frozen tissue has spread 2 mm out from the base of the lesion. Depending on size, this usually takes 5 to 10 seconds.
Repeat once if necessary.

Precautions

(1) Take great care with lesions on the faces of children and with pigmented skins. Hypopigmentation and hyperpigmentation can occur.

(2) Treat only if the diagnosis is certain: a confirmatory biopsy may be needed before treatment—as in Bowen's disease.

(3) Warn that a haemorrhagic blister may form at the site within 24 hours. This tendency can be reduced by a single application of a highly potent corticosteroid ointment immediately after treatment. Should a blister form it will remain for several days. If it is painful a sterile needle may be used to burst it and then a dry dressing can be applied.

(4) It may be unwise to treat lesions on both hands or feet at the same visit.

Electrocautery

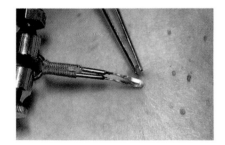

A heated element is used to coagulate the lesions. As no current passes through the body this is a safe procedure.

Common indications include (*a*) the removal of benign epidermal pedunculated tumours, such as skin tags; and (*b*) the destruction of small vascular lesions such as spider naevi. Only lesions that need no histological confirmation should be treated. Other indications for this procedure lie outside the scope of this article. There are two modes of cautery—shave cautery and pinpoint cautery.

Shave cautery is used on skin tags over 1 cm long. The correct attachment is needed. Pick up the skin tag with forceps and slice across the base with the cautery instrument. Local anaesthetic may be required.

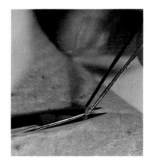

Equally well tolerated is touching a skin tag with the needle or ball point tip directly. The lesion mummifies immediately and drops off in 10 days.

Smaller lesions may be simply snipped off.

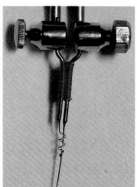

Pinpoint cautery attachment.

Blanch the lesion to identify feeding vessels. Then insert needle into feeding vessels in the cold state.

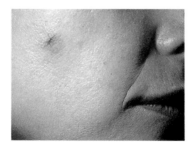

Spider naevus.

Pinpoint cautery is used on lesions such as spider naevi. A pinpoint attachment is needed. Locate the feeding vessel by blanching with a glass slide. Accurately position the needle element in the cold state into the lesion and apply current for less than 1 second. Warn the patient that a small scab will develop and fall off within 10 days. A local anaesthetic is seldom needed.

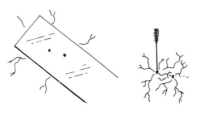

AUTOIMMUNITY AND SKIN DISEASE

Hypersensitivity

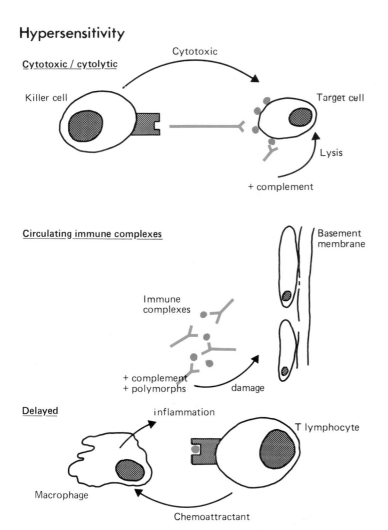

Autoimmunity is the state where the normal mechanisms of tolerance to self antigens are broken down. Autoantibodies and autoantigen specific T lymphocytes develop.

Autoantibodies may be produced against an organ specific antigen—for example, bullous pemphigoid antigen—or against a very widely distributed antigen such as DNA, as in lupus erythematosus. Not surprisingly, the resulting disease can be organ specific or non-organ specific. The pathogenesis is complex. It is not simply the effect of T lymphocytes locking on to autoantibody coated target cells with subsequent cell death ("cytotoxic" hypersensitivity); damage due to the deposition of circulating immune complexes; or, in some instances, cell mediated ("delayed") hypersensitivity related to specifically sensitised T cells. Defects in the control of immunological tolerance by T suppressor cells are now thought to be implicated as well.

Autoimmune diseases often run in families. Individuals with certain human leucocyte antigen (HLA) haplotypes are well known to be at risk of developing Hashimoto's thyroiditis or pernicious anaemia, and the same is true for systemic lupus erythematosus and pemphigus.

The skin reflects the range of autoimmune disease

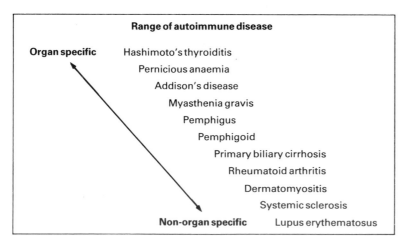

The skin is often an indicator of internal conditions, and autoimmunity is no exception. Pigmentation accompanies some organ specific disorders, such as Hashimoto's thyroiditis, Addison's disease, and primary biliary cirrhosis. A lemon yellow hue and canities occur with pernicious anaemia, and vitiligo like lesions and alopecia areata may be found in individuals with various autoimmune problems.

Non-organ specific autoimmune diseases often have prominent skin disease—for example, lupus erythematosus, systemic sclerosis, and dermatomyositis—but there are cutaneous organ specific disorders, principally pemphigus and pemphigoid.

Pemphigoid

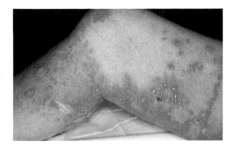

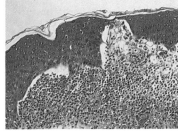

Split at dermatoepidermal junction.

Usually a condition of the elderly with a slight preponderance among women, bullous pemphigoid is characterised by large tense blisters arising on erythematous or normal looking skin. The limbs, trunk, and flexures are commonly affected; mouth lesions occur in 10% of patients. The disease responds readily to modest doses of oral prednisolone, and spontaneous remission is seen in up to a half of subjects, although relapses may occur.

Direct immunofluorescence

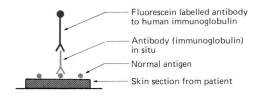

— Fluorescein labelled antibody to human immunoglobulin

— Antibody (immunoglobulin) in situ

— Normal antigen

— Skin section from patient

Indirect immunofluorescence

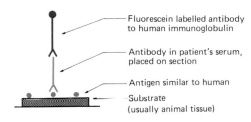

— Fluorescein labelled antibody to human immunoglobulin

— Antibody in patient's serum, placed on section

— Antigen similar to human

— Substrate (usually animal tissue)

Histologically, the blisters are subepidermal. Most patients have antibodies directed against the basement membrane zone circulating in their blood. These antibodies, usually of the IgG type, may be identified in serum by the *indirect* immunofluorescence method. This uses a tissue substrate (animal or sometimes human skin) cut freshly as a thin section on a slide, on to which the patient's serum is applied; the antibodies which attach to the basement membrane zone are shown by subsequently applying an antihuman immunoglobulin antibody which has been tagged with fluorescein, so that it shows up when the slide is visualised under ultraviolet radiation. The anti-basement membrane zone antibodies can be shown in a patient's perilesional skin by *direct* immunofluorescence. A freshly cut section of skin is reacted with a fluorescein labelled antibody to human IgG, and the deposited IgG can be seen as a continuous band at the basement membrane zone. The anti-BMZ antibodies are directed against bullous pemphigoid antigen, located in the lamina lucida of the basement membrane zone, and synthesised by the basal cells of the epidermis.

Other types of pemphigoid, such as cicatricial (which affects the ocular or oral membranes) or "localised" (often affecting a limited area on the head or neck), show similar histological and immunofluorescence profiles, although circulating anti-basement membrane zone antibodies are less commonly found. The same applies for pemphigoid ("herpes") gestationis, a rare but characteristic bullous eruption of pregnancy.

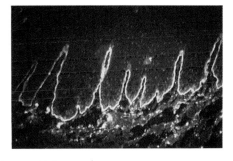

Indirect immunofluorescence.

Pemphigus

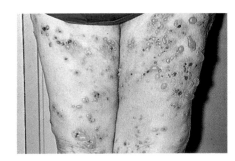

Less common than pemphigoid and more likely to prove fatal, pemphigus vulgaris is a disease of middle life. Oral lesions signal the onset in half of the patients and often precede cutaneous disease by months. Fragile superficial blisters develop over the scalp, face, back, chest, and flexures: the bullous element may not be apparent and lesions may consist of crusted erosions. Unlike with pemphigoid, high doses of prednisolone (often with other immunosuppressive agents) are required and spontaneous remission is exceptional.

The blister is intraepidermal. Ninety per cent of patients have circulating autoantibodies, IgG in type, directed against an intercellular substance of the epidermis and identifiable by indirect immunofluorescence. The levels of these antibodies correlate with disease activity, and evidence suggests that the antibodies produce the intraepidermal split. Direct immunofluorescence shows IgG antibodies deposited on the intercellular substance of the suprabasal epidermis in almost all patients. The antigen responsible has not yet been characterised.

Autoimmunity and skin disease

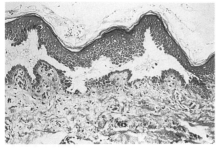

Intraepidermal split.

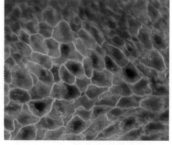

Direct immunofluorescence.

Other variants of pemphigus exist. Pemphigus vegetans gives hypertrophic, papillomatous lesions, whereas pemphigus foliaceus is characterised by shallow erosions on the face and scalp, and pemphigus erythematosus has some features of lupus erythematosus. Pemphigus is sometimes associated with myasthenia gravis, another organ specific autoimmune disease. Treatment with penicillamine can induce pemphigus: the eruption usually resolves when treatment with the drug is stopped.

Alopecia areata and vitiligo

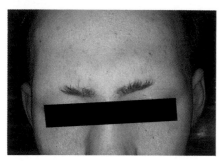

Alopecia areata.

Organ specific autoimmune diseases are more prevalent than expected in patients with both vitiligo and alopecia areata, and afflicted patients have an increased prevalence of organ specific autoantibodies. Despite these associations, however, no direct evidence implicates alopecia areata or vitiligo as an autoimmune disease.

Lupus erythematosus

Clinical variants of lupus erythematosus

Systemic
Subacute cutaneous
Discoid
(Neonatal)

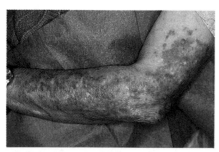

Subacute lupus erythematosus.

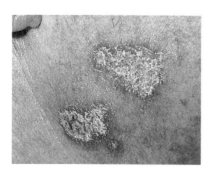

Discoid lupus erythematosus.

Discoid lupus erythematosus and systemic lupus erythematosus seem to be variants of the same disease, although only about 5% of those with the discoid type progress to systemic disease. A variety of autoantibodies to nuclear, nucleolar, and cytoplasmic antigens are found in lupus erythematosus. Almost 90% of patients with systemic lupus erythematosus have circulating antinuclear antibodies, but only a third of those with discoid lupus erythematosus show circulating antibodies.

Three quarters of patients with systemic lupus erythematosus have cutaneous disease. The "butterfly" eruption over the face is well known, but other cutaneous signs include photosensitivity, discoid lesions, alopecia, and vasculitis. A diagnosis of systemic lupus erythematosus requires the demonstration of multisystem disease with serological or haematological abnormalities. In addition to circulating antibodies, direct immunofluorescence of skin where there are no lesions may show granular deposition of various immunoglobulins and complement components at the dermoepidermal junction, the "lupus band" test.

In discoid lupus erythematosus, the discoid lesions typically occur in areas exposed to light, usually on the face. Circulating antinuclear antibodies and systemic symptoms are infrequent, although the "lupus band" test may be positive in lesional skin.

Patients with "subacute cutaneous" lupus erythematosus have a distinctive annular eruption, often with systemic (but not renal) disease, and usually show circulating antibodies to a cytoplasmic RNA nucleotide (Ro). Anti-Ro antibodies are similarly found in neonatal lupus erythematosus, which also has definitive skin signs.

Lupus erythematosus is often thought of as an immune complex disease with defects in T suppressor cell function. Ultraviolet radiation may generate antigenic nuclear products in the skin, with the development of clinical disease.

Dermatomyositis

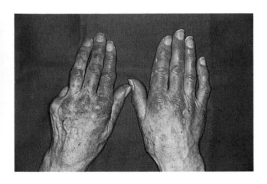

The dermatomyositis-polymyositis complex is a heterogeneous group of disorders with varying involvement of skin and muscle. Associations with malignancy, particularly in men aged over 40, and connective tissue disease, especially rheumatoid arthritis and systemic lupus erythematosus, represent distinct subtypes.

The purplish red heliotrope erythema around the eyelids, cheeks, and forehead, often with oedema, is typical. Bluish red scaly plaques on the dorsal aspects of the fingers and hands (especially over the joints) and nail fold telangiectasia are other features, although the eruption can be widespread.

Abnormalities of humoral and cellular immunity suggest an autoimmune cause. Although not specific, antibodies to skeletal muscle are found, and lymphocytes from affected patients show enhanced transformation on exposure to muscle antigens. Deposits of IgG, IgM, or C3 are described in skeletal muscle blood vessels on direct immunofluorescence, and IgG or IgM may be seen in the upper dermis. Antinuclear antibodies are present in the serum of some subjects.

Systemic sclerosis and morphoea

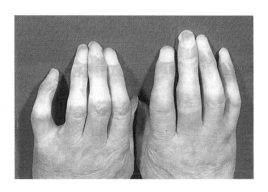

Morphoea, localised plaques or bands of sclerotic skin, is clinically distinct from systemic sclerosis, though histologically the skin changes are similar. Morphoea is a local form of systemic sclerosis, but affected patients lack the serological characteristics of the latter, and internal disease is uncommon or mild.

Skin changes are prominent in systemic sclerosis. Raynaud's phenomenon is almost invariable: the skin of the hands and forearms becomes tight and waxy, with atrophy of the finger pulp and flexion deformities. Telangiectasia, with radial furrowing around the mouth and restricted mouth opening, are characteristic. Disease of internal organs must be expected.

Almost all patients with systemic sclerosis have antibodies to nuclear or cytoplasmic antigens in their sera. Endothelial cell damage, related to humoral or T cell derived factors, may initiate a cascade of inflammation which results in fibrosis and sclerosis of the target organ.

Graft versus host disease

Graft versus host disease occurs after bone marrow transplantation, when immunocompetent cells of the graft react against the histoincompatible tissues of the immunosuppressed recipient. Acute and chronic forms are recognised, with cutaneous changes including a morbilliform eruption, toxic epidermal necrolysis, a lichen planus like eruption, and a scleroderma like syndrome.

THE SKIN AND SYSTEMIC DISEASE

When a man has on the skin of his body a swelling or an eruption or a spot . . . and the disease appears to be deeper than the skin it is a leprous disease.

Leviticus 13:2-3

Although arguments continue about what the Old Testament writers understood by "leprous," there was clearly an appreciation of the connection between the skin and systemic illness. As in ancient times, clinical signs in the skin may give valuable diagnostic clues to underlying disease. Sometimes the same condition affects both the skin and other organs, or severe skin disease itself may be the cause of generalised illness.

The skin is also a common target organ for allergic reactions to drugs, with a rash being the first clinical sign. The florid skin lesions of the acquired immune deficiency syndrome (AIDS) illustrate the results of infections when the immune response is impaired.

The cutaneous signs of systemic disease is a very large subject, on which much has been written, so a skin eruption that might indicate systemic disease is good reason to consult the large textbooks. Nevertheless, it is possible to give an outline of the more common skin changes that may be associated with systemic illness.

Erythematous rashes

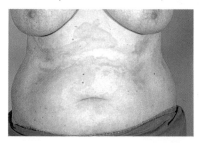

Rash from penicillin.

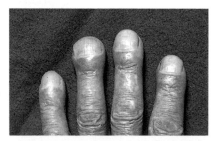

Erythema multiforme.

Allergic reactions to drugs, commonly the penicillins. There may be a widespread rash developing from a few days to two weeks after treatment with moderate illness (type III) or an acute life threatening anaphylactic reaction (types I and III) with acute angio-oedema and renal failure.

Infection—The characteristic rash of the various viral infections is, in a broad sense, also an allergic response. Less specific reactions such as erythema multiforme are commonly associated with infection—for example, herpes and other viral infections and streptococcal infection—but also with connective tissue disease and drugs such as sulphonamides.

In *carcinoid and phaeochromocytoma* vasoactive substances cause episodes of flushing and telangectasia.

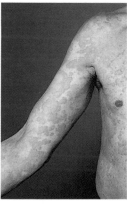

Figurate erythema.

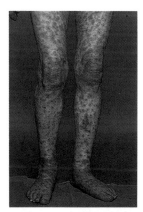

Erythema of nailbeds.

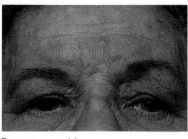

Dermatomyositis.

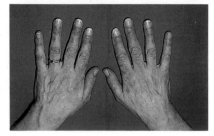

Neoplasia—Numerous patterns of widespread erythema have been described—the "*figurate erythemas*"—which may be associated with underlying carcinoma. *Dermatomyositis*, also a rare condition, has very high association in adults with underlying carcinoma commonly of the breasts, lung, ovary, or gastrointestinal tract. It is characterised by localised erythema with a purple hue, predominantly on the eyelids, cheeks and forehead. There may be similar changes on the dorsal surface of the fingers often with dilated nail fold capillaries. These changes may precede the discovery of an underlying tumour and may also fade away once it is removed. There is variable association with muscle aching and weakness.

Erythema of the nailbeds may be associated with connective tissue disease—such as lupus erythematosus, scleroderma, and dermatomyositis. "Clubbing" of the fingers may be associated.

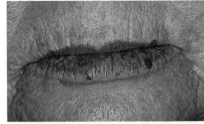

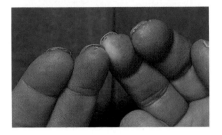

CRST syndrome.

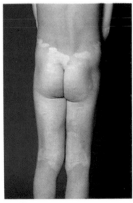

Vasculitis.

Telangiectasia and clubbing may be features of scleroderma in the CRST (Calcinosis, Raynaud's phenomenon, Scleroderma, and Telangiectasia) syndrome.

Erythrocyanosis is a dusky, red, cyanotic change in the skin over the legs and thighs, where there is a deep layer of underlying fat. The condition becomes worse in the winter months. It is most common in young women and usually resolves over the years. Lupus erythematosus, sarcoidosis, and tuberculous infection may localise in affected areas.

Livedo reticularis is a cyanotic, net-like discoloration of the skin over the legs. It may be idiopathic or associated with arteritis or changes in blood viscosity.

Spider naevi, which show a central blood vessel with radiating branches, are frequently seen in women (especially during pregnancy) and children. If they occur in large numbers, particularly in men, they may indicate liver failure. Palmar erythema and yellow nails may also be present.

Vasculitis and purpura of the skin may be associated with disease of the kidneys and other organs, as has already been discussed. "Splinter haemorrhages" under the nails are usually the result of minor trauma but may be associated with a wide range of conditions, including subacute bacterial endocarditis and rheumatoid arthritis.

Changes in pigmentation

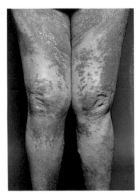

Vitiligo.

Autoimmune associations with vitiligo

Thyroid disease	Myasthenia gravis
Pernicious anaemia	Alopecia areata
Hypoparathyroidism	Halo naevus
Addison's disease	Morphoea and
Diabetes	lichen sclerosus

Hypopigmentation

A widespread partial loss of melanocyte functions with loss of skin colour is seen in hypopituitarism and is caused by an absence of melanocyte stimulating hormone. In the various types of autosomal recessive albinism there is a very considerable loss of pigment from the skin, hair, and eyes.

Localised depigmentation is most commonly seen in vitiligo, in which a family history of the condition is found in one third of the patients. In the sharply demarcated, symmetrical macular lesions there is loss of melanocytes and melanin. There is an increased incidence of organ specific antibodies and their associated diseases (table).

Other causes of hypopigmented macules include: postinflammatory conditions following psoriasis, eczema, lichen planus, and lupus erythematosus; infections—for example, tinea versicolor and leprosy; chemicals, such as hydroquinones, hydroxychloroquine, and arsenicals; reactions to pigmented naevi, seen in halo naevus; and genetic diseases, such as tuberous sclerosis ("ash leaf" macules).

The skin and systemic disease

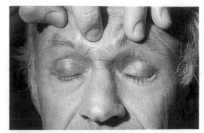

Argyria (silver salts in skin).

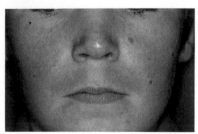

Melasma.

Hyperpigmentation

There is wide variation in the pattern of normal pigmentation as a result of heredity and exposure to the sun. Darkening of the skin may be due to an increase in the normal pigment melanin or to the deposition of bile salts in liver disease, iron salts (haemochromatosis), drugs, or metallic salts from ingestion.

Causes of hyperpigmentation include the following.

Hormonal—An increase in circulating hormones that have a melanocyte stimulating activity occurs in hyperthyroidism, Addison's disease, and acromegaly. In women who are pregnant or taking oral contraceptives there may be an increase in melanocytic pigmentation of the face. This is known as melasma (or chloasma) and occurs mainly on the forehead and cheeks. It may fade slowly. Sometimes a premenstrual darkening of the face occurs.

Increased deposition of haemosiderin is generalised in haemochromatosis. Localised red-brown discoloration of the legs is seen with longstanding varicose veins. It also occurs in a specific localised pattern in Schamberg's disease, when there is a "cayenne pepper" appearance of the legs and thighs.

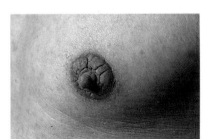

Acanthosis nigricans.

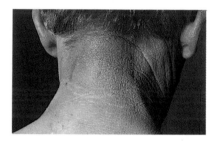

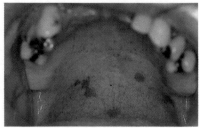

Pseudoacanthosis nigricans.

Neoplasia—Lymphomas may be associated with increased pigmentation. *Acanthosis nigricans*, characterised by darkening and thickening of the skin of the axillae, neck, nipples, and umbilicus, occurs with internal cancers, usually adenocarcinoma of the stomach. There is also a benign juvenile type. *Pseudo acanthosis nigricans* is much more common, consisting of simple darkening of the skin in the flexures of obese individuals; it is not associated with malignancy.

Drugs—Chlorpromazine and other phenothiazines may cause an increased pigmentation in areas exposed to the sun. Phenytoin can cause local hyperpigmentation of the face and neck.

Inflammatory reactions—Post inflammatory pigmentation is common, often following acute eczema, fixed drug eruptions, or lichen planus. Areas of lichenification from rubbing the skin are commonly darkened.

Malabsorption and deficiency states—In malabsorption syndromes, pellagra, and scurvy there is often frequently increased skin pigmentation.

Congenital conditions—There is clearly a marked variation in pigmentation and in the number of freckles in normal individuals. There may be localised well defined pigmented areas in neurofibromatosis with "cafe au lait" patches. Increased pigmentation with a blue tinge occurs over the lumbosacral region in the condition known as Mongolian blue spot.

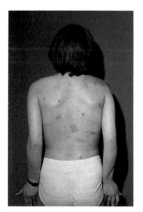

Neurofibromatosis.

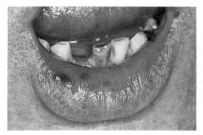

Peutz-Jeghers syndrome.

Peutz-Jeghers syndrome is inherited as an autosomal dominant characterised by pigmented macules of the oral mucosal membranes, lips, and face that appear in infancy. Benign intestinal polyps, mainly in the ileum and jejunum, which very rarely become malignant, are associated with the condition.

Malignant lesions

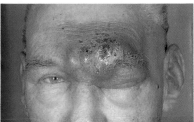
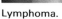
Lymphoma.

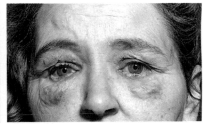
B cell lymphoma.

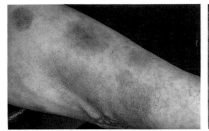
Mycosis fungoides.

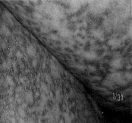
Poikiloderma.

Malignant lesions may cause skin changes such as acanthosis nigricans and dermatomyositis or produce secondary lesions. Lymphomas can arise in or invade the skin and pruritus may be associated with Hodgkin's disease.

Mycosis fungoides is a T cell lymphoma of cutaneous origin. Initially well demarcated erythematous plaques develop on covered areas with intense itching. In many cases there is a gradual progression to infiltrated lesions, nodules, and ulceration. In others the tumour may occur de novo or be preceded by generalised erythema.

Poikiloderma, in which there is telangiectasia, reticulate pigmentation, atrophy, and loss of pigment, may precede mycosis fungoides, but it is also seen after radiotherapy and in connective tissue diseases.

Parapsoriasis is a term used to cover maculopapular erythematous lesions that occur in middle and old age. Some cases undoubtedly develop into mycosis fungoides and a biopsy specimen should be taken of any such fixed plaques that do not clear with topical steroids.

The gut and the skin

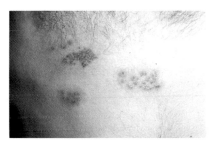
Early pyoderma gangrenosum.

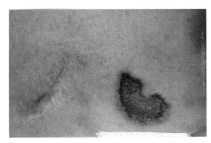
Pyoderma gangrenosum.

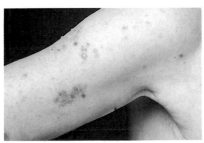
Dermatitis herpetiformis.

Vasculitis of various kinds, periarteritis nodosa, connective tissue diseases such as scleroderma, and many metabolic diseases produce both cutaneous and gastrointestinal lesions. There are, however, some specific associations.

Dry skin, asteatosis, and itching, with superficial eczematous changes and a "crazy paving" pattern, occur in malabsorption and cachectic states. Increased pigmentation, brittle hair and nails may also be associated.

Pyoderma gangrenosum—An area of non-specific inflammation and pustules breaks down to form a necrotic ulcer with hypertrophic margins. There is an underlying vasculitis. There is a strong association with ulcerative colitis and also with Crohn's disease, rheumatoid arthritis, and other diseases with an altered immune response.

Dermatitis herpetiformis, which has already been discussed, is an intensely itching, chronic disorder with erythematous and blistering lesions on the trunk and limbs. It is more common in men than women. Most patients have a gluten sensitive enteropathy with some degree of villus atrophy. There is an associated risk of small bowel lymphoma.

Other conditions—Peutz-Jeghers syndrome, with intestinal polyposis, has already been mentioned, but there are other rare congenital disorders with connective tissue and vascular abnormalities that affect the gut, such as Ehlers-Danlos syndrome and pseudoxanthoma elasticum (arterial gastrointestinal bleeding), purpuric vasculitis (bleeding from gastrointestinal lesions), and neurofibromatosis (intestinal neurofibromas).

Crohn's disease (regional ileitis)—Perianal lesions and sinus formation in the abdominal wall often occur. Glossitis and thickening of the lips and oral mucosa and vasculitis may be associated.

The skin and systemic disease
Diabetes and the skin

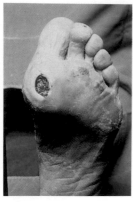
Diabetic ulcer.

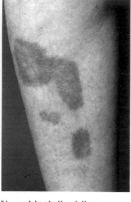
Necrobiosis lipoidica.

In diabetes the disturbances of carbohydrate-lipid metabolism, small blood vessel lesions, and neural involvement may be associated with skin lesions. The more common of these include the following.

Infection—Diabetics have an increased susceptibility to staphylococcal, coliform, and pseudomonal infection. *Candida albicans* infection is also more common in diabetics.

Vascular lesions—"Diabetic dermopathy," due to a microangiopathy, consists of erythematous papules which slowly resolve to leave a scaling macule on the limbs. Atherosclerosis with impaired peripheral circulation is often associated with diabetes.

Ulceration due to neuropathy (trophic ulcers) or impaired blood supply may occur, particularly on the feet.

Specific skin lesions

Necrobiosis lipoidica—40-60% of patients with this condition may develop diabetes but it is not very common in diabetics (0·3%). As the name indicates, there is necrosis of the connective tissue with lymphocytic and granulomatous infiltrate. There is replacement of degenerating collagen fibres with lipid material. It usually occurs over the shin but may appear at any site.

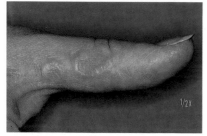
Granuloma annulare.

Granuloma annulare usually presents with localised papular lesions on the hands and feet but may occur elsewhere. The lesions may be partly or wholly annular and may be single or multiple. There is some degree of necrobiosis with histiocytes forming "palisades" as well as giant cells and lymphocytes. It is seen more commonly in women, usually those aged under 30. There is an association with insulin dependent diabetes. In itself it is a harmless and self limiting condition that slowly clears but may recur.

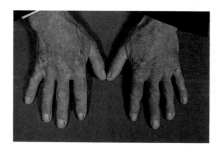
Porphyria.

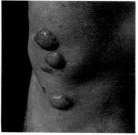
Xanthomas.

Other metabolic diseases may cause skin change—for example, the xanthomas of hyperlipidaemia and photosensitivity with blistering in porphyria.

Other conditions

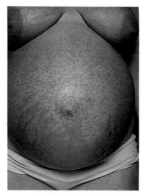
Polymorphic eruption.

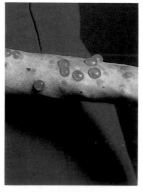
Pemphigoid gestationis.

Pregnancy may be associated with pruritus, in which the skin appears normal in 15-20% of women. Less commonly a blistering disorder known as pemphigoid gestationis is seen. An itching polymorphic eruption of pregnancy, which is more common, may represent a less severe form. It usually occurs in the third trimester on the abdomen and then becomes widespread. There may be a postpartum exacerbation before it resolves.

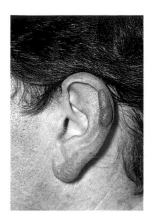
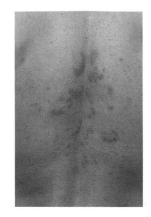

Sarcoidosis of the skin appears in various forms—as papules, nodules, plaques, or large cyanotic lesions ("lupus pernio"). Erythema nodosum may be associated.

Thyroid disease

Hypothyroidism	Hyperthyroidism
Dry skin	Soft, thickened skin
Oedema of eyelids and hands	Pretibial myxoedema
Absence of sweating	Increased sweating
Coarse, thin hair—loss of pubic, axillary, and eyebrow hair	(palms and soles)
	Thinning of scalp hair
Pale "ivory" skin	Diffuse pigmentation
Brittle poorly growing nails	Rapidly growing nails
Purpura, bruising, and telangiectasia	Palmar erythema
	Facial flushing

Thyroid disease is associated with changes in the skin, which may sometimes be the first clinical signs. There may be evidence of the effect of altered concentrations of thyroxine on the skin, with changes in texture and hair growth. Associated increases in thyroid stimulating hormone concentration may lead to pretibial myxoedema. In autoimmune thyroid disease vitiligo and other autoimmune conditions may be present.

ACKNOWLEDGMENTS

Many colleagues have made useful comments on the ABC of Dermatology articles and, where appropriate, changes have accordingly been made to the text. In some cases, however, the points raised related to specialised or controversial aspects which could not be discussed at length within the limits of an ABC.

I am grateful to Dr Peter Ball, consultant in infectious diseases, Fife Health Board, for comments on infectious diseases, Dr M Jones, consultant in infectious diseases, City Hospital, Edinburgh, for comments on parvovirus infections, and Mr C V Ruckley, consultant surgeon, Royal Infirmary, Edinburgh, for comments on varicose ulcers.

Most of the illustrations are from the collection at the Victoria Hospital, Kirkcaldy, thanks to the expertise of Mr W McIntyre and his staff. Some are from the collection at the Royal Infirmary, Edinburgh, and a few were taken by the author.

The following colleagues kindly provided illustrations of specific conditions: Dr Peter Ball, rubella; Dr D H H Robertson, genital herpes; Mr C V Ruckley, varicose veins; Dr G B Colver, spider naevus.

P K B
May 1988

INDEX

Index

Index